KV-034-509

Speak Spanish Now for Medical Professionals

HS 468 JONES

Speak Spanish Now for Medical Professionals

A Customized Learning Approach for Doctors, Nurses, Nursing and Medical Assistants

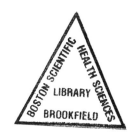

Brian K. Jones

Carolina Academic Press

Durham, North Carolina

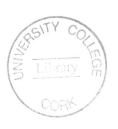

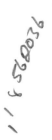

Copyright © 2007
Brian K. Jones
All Rights Reserved.

Library of Congress Cataloging-in-Publication Data

Jones, Brian K. (Brian Keith), 1971-
  Speak Spanish now for medical professionals / by Brian K. Jones.
    p. cm.
  Includes bibliographical references and index.
  ISBN 978-1-59460-318-1 (alk. paper)
  1. Spanish language--Conversation and phrase books (for medical
personnel) I. Title.

  PC4120.M3J66 2007
  468.3'42102461--dc22   2007021261

Carolina Academic Press
700 Kent Street
Durham, North Carolina
Tel: (919) 489-7468
Fax: (919) 493-5668
www.cap-press.com

Printed in the United States of America.

Contents

A Customized Learning Approach to Language

The purpose of this text is to assist those in the medical profession with effective, immediate communication with Spanish-speaking patients. Therefore, this book's approach is to teach straightforward, oral communication that requires the learner to verbally produce while relying little on listening skills. It is intended primarily as one-way communication and does not require the learning of grammar or the development of written communique. However, certain anticipated responses have been included for you. Even if the speaker does not use the exact answer, you will be able to recognize fragments and then take control of the conversation. Upon successfully mastering the phrases of the text, the learner will be able to attend to the common needs of patients they encounter on a daily basis, explain to them routine procedures, ascertain patient information and interact with patients in a culturally sensitive manner.

Using This Text

This text has been designed to encompass four groups of medical professionals: doctors, nurses, nursing and medical assistants. This is not to say that other professionals in the medical community will not find this text practical, however, the focus is on those persons who would find themselves interacting most with the patient. Furthermore, not all sections of the text may be specific to each group's job duties. The text allows you to pick and choose what you will learn and concentrate on those areas that are most beneficial to you and your respective medical profession. The pages have been perforated so you can easily remove sections you will not use in order to customize the book or make the most used pages more portable. The options are left open to you.

In learning the words and phrases in this text, you will be concentrating on oral communication. You will only write in Spanish when preparing notecards or preparing phrases to be used during an activity unless your curriculum requires it. Grammatical explanations are not necessary for any of the information you will be learning. Your instructor will lead you through a wide variety of communicative exercises that will help you internalize these phrases and their meanings and get away from the daunting task of rote memorization. The accompanying CD will enable you to listen to the phrases and practice their pronunciation. Your instructor may also choose to provide you with strategies that will make the CD more beneficial to you as a study aid. The CD may be used in class but is also highly recommended as an independent study aid.

The sections have been designated titles to help you manage the selection of the material you will choose to learn. However, make sure to glance through all of them for miscellaneous phrases you may find beneficial in your interactions with Hispanic patients. Feel free to mix and match phrases from various sections in order to tailor the information you will need to convey to and/or obtain from your patients. Most of the time, the phrases follow a logical order for their delivery. However, there is no prescribed order that must be followed each time they are used.

Immediately before each set of phrases, when appropriate, you will find a section titled BEFORE YOU BEGIN. These sections present pertinent information that will enable health care professionals to better understand the cultural differences between Hispanic and American patients and be able to provide them with an atmosphere more conducive to the doctor/patient rapport with which they are most comfortable. Current statistics and important health-related information that focuses on the Hispanic population have been included.

Finally, at the end of most chapters, you will find a NOTES section followed by a PRACTICAL ACTIVITIES section that includes activities and specific questions about the respective chapter and its content. Where applicable, an optional cyber-investigation exercise (Internet search activity) meant to build upon cultural information presented in the BEFORE YOU BEGIN section has been included.

Pronunciation

The purpose of the pronunciation patterns found directly above each Spanish phrase is to immediately generate proper or nearly proper pronunciation. By following these easy guidelines, communication becomes instantaneous. The words and sounds used in the pronunciation patterns are based on those used in English, so say what you see. Practice exercises to aid you in interpreting the pronunciation patterns and to prepare you for making those sounds correctly follow these brief explanations. Be sure to follow them in the prescribed order.

Instructions for reading the pronunciation patterns:

1. The separation of words has been indicated by one or more spaces. Example:

   bway-*nohs* *dee*-*ahs*. (two word phrase)
   Buenos días.

2. The separation of syllables has been indicated by a *hyphen*. Example:

   bway-*nohs* *dee*-*ahs*. (both words have two syllables)
   Buenos días.

3. Syllables written in *bolded letters* are emphasized when spoken. Example:

   bway-*nohs* *dee*-*ahs*. (emphasis on **bway** and **dee**)
   Buenos días.

4. Syllables written in *unbolded letters* are not emphasized. Example:

   bway-*nohs* *dee*-*ahs*. (no emphasis on -nohs and -ahs)
   Buenos días.

5. The *upward pointing arrow*, or the (^) sign, indicates a combination of sounds to be pronounced as one (1) syllable. Example:

   grah-*see^ahs*. *(see^ahs is one sound)*
   Gracias.

6. The *double r* you will see indicates a rolled or trilled "r" sound. Example:

   rray-*goo*-*lahr*. (rr of *rray* is rolled/trilled)
   Regular.

The double r, or "rr" in Spanish, is represented by "rr" in the pronunciation key. Do the best you can to imitate the sound but do not get frustrated, as long as you are making the effort you will be understood. Keep practicing and it will come with time. Likewise, anyone who has any prior knowledge of Spanish pronunciation may know that the *Spanish v* is often pronounced as a soft *English b*, although some dialects of spoken Spanish do pronounce the *Spanish v* the same as the *English v*. However, for the sake of consistency and simplicity, the *Span-*

ish v has been represented as the *letter b* in the pronunciation patterns throughout the text and may be pronounced as such.

Introductory Exercise: With a partner or as a group, randomly select phrases from the text, analyze them and identify each of the above elements of the **pronunciation** patterns. Do not practice pronunciation yet. Just become familiar with how to interpret the **pronunciation** patterns. **You must practice the pronunciation exercises thoroughly before attempting to read the pronunciation patterns for the phrases!**

Lingual Aerobics (so to speak) . . .

Getting started: Just like any other muscle in your body that is not accustomed to certain motions and actions, the tongue and mouth are no different. These exercises will help you warm up these muscles and form the correct positions with you mouth and tongue to produce relatively authentic Spanish pronunciation from the very beginning.

Pronunciation Exercise 1: This oral exercise is to help you become used to the basic sounds you will use and see throughout this text, all of which are based on the five basic vowel sounds of the Spanish alphabet - A, E, I, O, U. Though they are the same five vowels found in English, their sounds are rather different. In order to facilitate their production, in practicing this exercise, say exactly what you see as you would in English. Start by saying the words and sounds, going column by column (in sequence according to numbers) together as a group, then row by row, individually, small group, pairs, etc. Remember, the sounds **bolded** in the first column should be applied to the combinations you will practice in each column that follows. These bolded sounds are the actual sounds of the corresponding Spanish vowel.

Spanish Vowel	#1	#2	#3	#4	#5	#6	#7	#8	#9
A	*hah*	*ah*	*bah*	*kah*	*lah*	*mah*	*sah*	*tah*	*yah*
E	*day*	*ay*	*bay*	*kay*	*lay*	*may*	*say*	*tay*	*yay*
I	*see*	*ee*	*bee*	*kee*	*lee*	*mee*	*see*	*tee*	*yee*
O	*oh*	*oh*	*boh*	*koh*	*loh*	*moh*	*soh*	*toh*	*yoh*
U	*food*	*oo*	*boo*	*koo*	*loo*	*moo*	*soo*	*too*	*yoo*

Pronunciation Exercise 2: The second practice exercise builds upon the previous one by introducing you to sound combinations you will use and see throughout the text. Practice these in the same manner as the first set.

#1	#2	#3	#4	#5	#6
stah	*bway*	*tree*	*ahr*	*nahs*	*tahr*
chah	*stay*	*skree*	*ayr*	*nays*	*tayr*
grah	*pway*	*mwee*	*eer*	*nees*	*teer*
blah	*tray*	*ghee**	*ohr*	*nohs*	*tohr*
trah	*gway*	*flee*	*oor*	*noos*	*toor*

* This *g* is like the *g* sound in the word *get* but pronounced with the *long ee* sound.

Pronunciation Exercise 3: Starting with column 1, make sure to emphasize the bolded letters according to the pronunciation key. Beginning in column 4, start to incorporate the ^ sign indicating the combination of sounds pronounced as one syllable.

#1	#2	#3	#4
gah-nahs	ah-**sayr**	**tee**^ay-nay	nah-see-**mee**^ayn-toh
dohn-day	ay-spah-**nyohl**	**kee**^ay-rayn	sah-rahm-**pee**^ohn
pah-gahn	rray-spee-**rahr**	kee-**see**^ay-rah	dee^ah-**bay**-tays
ah-nyoh**	door-**meer**	ee-**stoh**-ree^ah	ee-payr-tayn-**see**^ohn
kwahn-toh	rray-say-**tahr**	**see**^ayn-toh	see-**ghee**^ayn-tay

  * This *g* is like the *g sound* in the word *get* but pronounced with the *long ee* sound.
** The *ny* is pronounced like the *ni* in the English word *onion*.

Pronunciation Exercise 4: Look through the text paying attention only to the pronunciation key and practice random examples as a class then in pairs.

Speak Spanish Now
for
Medical Professionals

Chapter 1

Breaking the Ice with Spanish-Speaking Patients: Greetings, Courtesy Expressions, and Goodbyes

Before You Begin

The Hispanic culture is a very respectful one full of customs and traditions. Regardless of a person's socioeconomic rank, the expectation of mutual respect still exists. Spanish speakers lean toward formality, even in their treatment of one another. As in American culture, a firm handshake is a common way of saying hello and goodbye. A common exchange of greetings between women, as well as men and women who are close friends or family, is a hug and a light kiss on a cheek.

The words and phrases you learn throughout this text exemplify the etiquette practiced by Hispanics. They are all appropriate for the environment in which you will use them and the interactions you will have with your Spanish-speaking clients. Lastly, three of the most important phrases you can learn are *gracias*, *por favor* and *de nada* (found in this section). Feel free to use them liberally, especially *por favor*, when making requests. You will be sure to generate an instant air of respect between any Spanish-speaker and yourself.

Phrases

English	Pronunciation & Spanish
1. Hello.	*oh-lah.* Hola.
2. Good morning.	*bway-nohs dee-ahs.* Buenos días.[1]
3. Good Afternoon.	*bway-nahs tahr-days.* Buenas tardes.[1]
4. Good evening. / Good night.	*bway-nahs noh-chays.* Buenas noches.[1]
5. Sir / Mr.	*say-nyohr.* Señor.
6. Ma'am / Mrs.	*say-nyoh-rah.* Señora.[2]
7. Miss / Ms.	*say-nyoh-ree-tah.* Señorita.[2]

BOSTON SCIENTIFIC HEALTH SCIENCES LIBRARY BROOKFIELD

3

8. How are you (today)?	*koh-moh ay-**stah** (oy)?* ¿Cómo está (hoy)?	
9. (Very) well. (And you?)	*(mwee) bee^ayn (ee oo-**stayd**?)* (Muy) bien. (Y Ud.?)³	
10. Okay.	*rray-goo-**lahr**.* Regular.	
11. Not too badly.	*ah-**see** ah-**see**.* Así, así.	
12. Not (very) well.	*(mwee) mahl.* (Muy) mal.⁴	
13. I'm sorry.	*loh **see^ayn**-toh.* Lo siento.	
14. Until later.	*ahs-tah **loo^ay**-goh.* Hasta luego.	
15. Goodbye.	*ah-**dee^ohs**.* Adiós.	
16. Thank you (very much).	*(**moo**-chahs) **grah**-see^ahs.* (Muchas) gracias.	
17. Please.	*pohr fah-**bohr**.* Por favor.	
18. You're welcome.	*day **nah**-dah.* De nada.	
19. Pardon. *[stating **excuse me** after an action]*	*payr-**dohn**.* Perdón.	
20. Excuse me. *[stating **excuse me** before an action]*	*kohn payr-**mee**-soh.* Con permiso.	
21. Okay. (Fine.)	*ay-**stah** bee^ayn.* Está bien.⁵	
22. Have a nice day.	*kay **pah**-say oon bwayn **dee**-ah.* Qué pase un buen día.	

Notes

¹ For simplicity's sake, use *Buenos días* from early morning (generally sun-up) to noon, *Buenas tardes* from noon to sundown and *Buenas noches* from sun-down to early morning. *Buenas noches* may be used as a greeting or a goodbye after sundown as well.

² Though a woman may not appear young, if she is not married, she is still a *Señorita*. Also, *señorita* is often abbreviated as *Srta.*, *señora* as *Sra.* and *señor* as *Sr.*

³ The word *usted* is commonly abbreviated as *Ud.* Whenever you see this abbreviation, make sure to say the entire word.

⁴ This phrase is a question of wellbeing and not one of a diagnostic nature, the literal translation of *muy mal* (very badly) is not implied.

⁵ This is very common for expressing agreement and comprehension. Another possible translation would be the English *alright*.

Practical Activities

A. Oral Practice

Instructions: With a partner, take turns responding in Spanish to each situation presented below only using phrases from this chapter. Try to implement as many alternative ways as possible to convey each situation.

1. Greet an unmarried older female patient and ask how she is doing.

2. Thank a male patient and say goodbye.

3. Respond to a married female patient who asks how you are doing and then ask how she is doing.

B. Matching

Instructions: Without looking back at the phrases presented in this chapter, try to match the English expression with its Spanish counterpart. Check your answers after you have finished.

1. ___ Pardon.	a. Muy mal.
2. ___ How are you today?	b. Hasta luego.
3. ___ Until later.	c. De nada.
4. ___ Okay.	d. Lo siento.
5. ___ Hello.	e. Muchas gracias.
6. ___ Not too bad.	f. Regular.
7. ___ Thank you very much.	g. Perdón.
8. ___ You're welcome.	h. Así, así.
9. ___ Not very well.	i. ¿Cómo está?
10. ___ I'm sorry.	j. Hola.

C. Short Answer Questions

Instructions: Answer the following questions based on information you learned in this chapter.

1. What are the general differences between the greetings *Buenos días, Buenas tardes* and *Buenas noches*?

2.   When would you address a female as *señora* and *señorita*?

Cyber-Investigation

Find a minimum of **four** additional Hispanic customs and/or traditions not mentioned in the **Before You Begin** section above. If applicable, discuss how they might possibly influence your relationship with Hispanic clients as a medical professional.

Chapter 2

General Administration

Section 1
Questions, Requests, and Responses

Before You Begin

Hispanic patients will have varying degrees of language skills, both in Spanish and English. Depending upon their level of education, they may be literate, semi-literate or illiterate in their native language. Likewise, depending upon the length of time they have spent in the United States, their knowledge of the English language will vary greatly. Since a deep sense of pride is innate to the Hispanic culture, it may be difficult to immediately recognize the abilities of the person with whom you are dealing. However, assess the situation as you interact with the patient with care and respect and be sure to avoid causing him or her any sense of shame or embarrassment.

Unlike many Americans who have a first, middle and last name, the majority of Hispanics have a first name followed by two surnames . These surnames consist first of the father's surname followed by the mother's maiden name. It is important to understand how to distinguish these components of a Hispanic name for the sake of alphabetizing documents, etc., Hispanic names are ordered according to the father's surname.

For example:

If *Sara **Montero*** and *Pedro **García*** have a child named *Miguel*, the child's complete name would be *Miguel **García Montero***.

His last name is technically ***García*** and would appear as such on documents. Likewise, he would be alphabetized under the letter ***G*** for ***García***.

Phrases

English	Pronunciation & Spanish
1. How can I help you?	*ayn kay **pway**-doh sayr-**beer**-lay?* ¿En qué puedo servirle?
2. I want to see a doctor.	***kee^ay**-roh bayr ah oon dohk-**tohr** / **oo**-nah dohk-**toh**-rah.* Quiero ver a un doctor / una doctora.[1]
3. I want to make an appointment.	***kee^ay**-roh ah-**sayr oo**-nah **see**-tah.* Quiero hacer una cita.
4. Do you speak English?	***ah**-blah een-**glays?*** ¿Habla inglés?
5. Yes.	*see.* Sí.

6. No.

noh.
No.

---

7. A little.

*oon **poh**-koh.*
Un poco.

---

8. I don't speak Spanish.

*noh **ah**-bloh ay-spah-**nyohl**.*
No hablo español.

---

9. I speak very little Spanish.

***ah**-bloh mwee **poh**-koh ay-spah-**nyohl**.*
Hablo muy poco español.

---

10. Do you know how to read and write?

***ah**-bay lay-**ayr** ee ay-skree-**beer**?*
¿Sabe leer y escribir?

---

11. Do you have an appointment?

***tee^ay**-nay **see**-tah?*
¿Tiene cita?

---

12. Would you like to see a doctor?

*kee-**see^ay**-rah bayr ah oon dohk-**tohr**?*
¿Quisiera ver a un doctor?

---

13. Is this your first appointment with us?

***ay**-stah ays soo pree-**may**-rah **see**-tah kohn noh-**soh**-trohs?*
¿Esta es su primera cita con nosotros?

---

14. What is your full name?

*kwahl ays soo **nohm**-bray kohm-**play**-toh?*
¿Cuál es su nombre completo?

---

15. Please repeat.

*rray-**pee**-tah, pohr fah-**bohr**.*
Repita, por favor.

---

16. Will you write it for me here?

*may loh ay-**skree**-bay ah-**kee**?*
¿Me lo escribe aquí?

---

17. Speak (more) slowly, please.

***ah**-blay (mahs) day-**spah**-see^oh pohr fah-**bohr**.*
Hable (más) despacio, por favor.

---

18. Who is your doctor?

***kee^ayn** ays soo dohk-**tohr** (dohk-**toh**-rah)?*
¿Quién es su doctor(a)?[1]

---

19. I'm sorry.

*loh **see^ayn**-toh.*
Lo siento.

---

20. I don't understand.

*noh kohm-**prayn**-doh.*
No comprendo.

---

21. Will you write your doctor's name

*ay-**skree**-bah ayl **nohm**-bray day soo dohk-**tohr** (dohk-**toh**-rah)*
Escriba el nombre de su doctor(a)

here for me, please.

*ah-**kee** pohr fah-**bohr**.*
aquí por favor.[1]

---

22. Write it here, please.

*ay-**skree**-bah-loh ah-**kee** pohr fah-**bohr**.*
Escríbalo aquí, por favor.

---

23. Fill out these forms, please.

***yay**-nay **ay**-stohs foor-moo-**lah**-ree^ohs pohr fah-**bohr**.*
Llene estos formularios, por favor.

---

24. Bring me the forms when you finish.

***trah^ee**-gah-may lohs foor-moo-**lah**-ree^ohs **kwahn**-doh tayr-**mee**-nay.*
Tráigame los formularios cuando termine.

D) Short Answer Questions

Instructions: Answer the following questions based on information you learned in this chapter.

1. When would you use *doctor* as opposed to *doctora*?

2. What are two other alternative terms for *doctor* and *doctora* you might hear?

3. Regarding Hispanic names, using your own first, middle and and last name, pair up with a classmate and apply the Hispanic method of surnames. Chart your names on a piece of paper to analyze how they evolve. Share your examples with other pairs to see how their names turned out.

Cyber-Investigation

As you have read above in **Before You Begin**, the level of education of the average Hispanic varies from that of the average American in the United States. Why do you think this to be the case? Find 3-4 pieces of data that support your beliefs. Other than reasons mentioned above, how might one's educational level affect their view of the importance of health care?

	feer-may ah-kee pohr fah-bohr
25. Sign here, please.	Firme aquí, por favor.
	pway-day ay-spay-rahr ayn lah sah-lah day ay-spay-rah.
26. You may wait in the waiting room.	Puede esperar en la sala de espera.
	lay yah-mahn ayn oon moh-mayn-toh.
27. They'll call you back in a moment.	Le llaman en un momento.
	oon moh-mayn-toh pohr fah-bohr.
28. Just a moment, please.	Un momento, por favor.
	day ah-kwayr-doh.
29. Okay.	De acuerdo.
	noh ah^ee proh-blay-mah.
30. No problem.	No hay problema.

Notes

[1] The word *doctor* refers to a male doctor whereas the word *doctora* refers to a female doctor. Unless you know, use *doctor* until the patient has specified. You may also hear or choose to use the terms *médico* (**may-dee-koh**) for a male doctor and *médica* **may-dee-kah)** for a female doctor.

Practical Activities I

A) Oral Practice

Instructions: Using only SPANISH, obtain the following information from a patient.

1. Ask if the patient speaks English and then state that you speak only a little Spanish.
2. Ask for the patient's complete name and if (s)he has an appointment.
3. Ask the patient to fill out the appropriate forms, bring them to you when completed, then to please wait in the waiting room.
4. Ask the patient to write down the doctor's name for you, sign in and then explain (s)he will be called in a moment.

B) Matching

Instructions: Without looking back at the phrases presented in this chapter, try to match the beginning fragment of each SPANISH phrase with its correct ending in order to complete the entire expression. Finally, add the correct punctuation (. or ?) at the end of the phrase indicating whether it is a question or a statement.

1. ___	¿Quién es . . .	a. su primera cita con nosotros
2. ___	¿Quisiera ver . . .	b. escribe aquí
3. ___	¿En qué . . .	c. una cita
4. ___	¿Me lo . . .	d. a un doctor
5. ___	¿Cuál es . . .	e. poco español
6. ___	Quiero hacer . . .	f. puedo servirle
7. ___	¿Esta es . . .	g. por favor
8. ___	Hablo muy . . .	h. su doctor
9. ___	Un momento,	i. su nombre completo
10. ___	Escríbalo . . .	j. aquí

C) Translation

Instructions: Write the meaning of the SPANISH phrases you matched above. '
and check your translation with the ENGLISH phrases provided in this chapter.

1. _____   6. _____

2. _____   7. _____

3. _____   8. _____

4. _____   9. _____

5. _____   10. _____

Section 2
Making Appointments and Scheduling Follow-up Visits

Before You Begin

In the Hispanic culture, the concept of time is relatively different. Punctualilty is not a great concern, and being late for events is considered socially acceptable. Therefore, if this is of great importance to your appointment scheduling make sure to reitierate office policies regarding scheduling with the appropriate phrases provided in this chapter.

Many countries, including Spanish-speaking ones, use a 24-hour clock instead of a 12-hour one. For example, 1 p.m. would be 13:00 where as 1 a.m. would be 1:00. Don't worry about learning the 24-hour clock. As long as you are clear about stating in the morning, in the afternoon, or in the evening, there should be no confusion. Also, a calendar in Spanish will start on Monday instead of Sunday.

Phrases

English	Pronunciation & Spanish
1. Do you need to make an appointment?	*nay-say-**see**-tah ah-**sayr** oo-nah **see**-tah?* ¿Necesita hacer una cita?
2. With whom?	*kohn kee^ayn?* ¿Con quién?
3. Which day do you prefer to come?	*ayn kay **dee**-ah pray-**fee**^**ay**-ray bay-**neer**?* ¿En qué día prefiere venir?[1]
4. What time do you prefer to come?	*ah kay **oh**-rah pray-**fee**^**ay**-ray vay-**neer**?* ¿A qué hora prefiere venir?[1]
5. I need to schedule your (follow-up)	*nay-say-**see**-toh ah-**sayr**-lay oo-nah* Necesito hacerle una
appointment.	***see**-tah (day say-ghee-**mee**^**ayn**-toh).* cita (de seguimiento).
6. You should return in . . .	***bwayl**-bah ayn . . .* Vuelva en . . .
one week.	***oo**-nah say-**may**-nah.* una semana.
two weeks.	*kah-**tohr**-say **dee**-ahs.* catorce días.
one month.	*oon mays.* un mes.
six months.	*says **may**-says.* seis meses.
one year.	*oon **ah**-nyoh.* un año.

7. Show me on the calendar

*een-**dee**-kay ayn ayl kah-layn-**dah**-ree^oh*
Indique en el calendario

   when you prefer to come back.

__kwahn__-doh pray-__fee^ay__-ray bay-__neer__.
cuándo prefiere venir.[1]

8. The office is closed . . .

ayl kohn-sool-__toh__-ree^oh ay-__stah__ say-__rrah__-do . . .
El consultorio está cerrado . . .

   that day.

__ay__-say __dee__-ah.
ese día.

   at that time.

ah __ay__-sah __oh__-rah.
a esa hora.

9. I'm going to confirm your appointment.

lay boy ah kohn-feer-__mahr__ lah __see__-tah.
Le voy a confirmar la cita.

10. Your appointment is . . .

soo __see__-tah ays . . .
Su cita es . . . [1]

   Monday

__loo__-nays
lunes

   Tuesday

__mahr__-tays
martes

   Wednesday

mee-__ayr__-koh-lays
miércoles

   Thursday

__whay__-bays
jueves

   Friday

__bee^ayr__-nays
viernes

   Saturday

__sah__-bah-doh
sábado

   at one

ah lah __oo__-nah
a la una

   at two

ah lahs dohs
a las dos

   at three

ah lahs trays
a las tres

   at four

ah lahs __kwah__-troh
a las cuatro

   at five

ah lahs __seen__-koh
a las cinco

   at six

ah lahs says
a las seis

   at seven

ah lahs __see^ay__-tay
a las siete

at eight	*ah lahs oh-choh* a las ocho
at nine	*ah lahs noo^ay-bay* a las nueve
at ten	*ah lahs dee^ays* a las diez
at eleven	*ah lahs ohn-say* a las once
at twelve	*ah lahs doh-say* a las doce
fifteen	*ee kwahr-toh* y cuarto
thirty	*ee may-dee^ah* y media
forty-five	*kwah-rayn-tah ee seen-koh* cuarenta y cinco
in the morning.	*day lah mah-nyay-nah.* de la mañana.
in the afternoon.	*day lah tahr-day.* de la tarde.
in the evening	*day lah noh-chay.* de la noche.

11. I'm calling on behalf of Dr._____	*yah-moh day pahr-tay dayl dohk-tohr / day lah dohk-toh-rah —.* Llamo de parte del doctor / de la doctora —.[2]

12. Is . . . available?	*ay- stah . . .* ¿Está . . .
Mr. — . . .	*ayl say-nyohr —?* el señor —?
Mrs. — . . .	*lah say-nyoh-rah —?* la señora —?
Ms. — . . .	*lah say-nyoh-ree-tah —?* la señorita —?

13. I need to confirm an appoinment for . . .	*nay-say-see-toh kohn-feer-mahr oo-nah see-tah pah-rah . . .* Necesito confirmar una cita para . . . [2]
Mr. — . . .	*ayl say-nyohr —?* el señor —?
Mrs. — . . .	*lah say-nyoh-rah —?* la señora —?
Ms. — . . .	*lah say-nyoh-ree-tah —?* la señorita —?

14. Will you still make it?	*pway-day bay-neer toh-dah-bee-ah?* Puede venir todavía?[2]
15. It is important to arrive on time.	*ays eem-pohr-tahn-tay yay-gahr ah tee^aym-poh.* Es importante legar a tiempo.
16. You will not be able to see the doctor	*noh poh-drah bayr ahl dohk-tohr* No podrá ver al doctor
if you arrive late.	*see yay-gah tahr-day.* si llega tarde.

Notes

[1] Using the overlay cards provided in the **Appendix** for this section, lay the name of the month and the days of the week over those of your desk calendar. Divide a sheet of paper into three columns, writing the numbers *1–12* in the first column, *:15 (cuarto), :30 (media), :45 (cuarenta y cinco)* in the second and *A.M.* and *P.M.* in the third one. Use these tools as your visual references to guide both you and the patient through the appointment-making process. Keep all of this handy for when you need to confirm appointments as well. Although there is a more complicated way to express *:45* when telling time, the strategy employed here is meant to be easier for an English speaker to grasp. Also, the word for Sunday, *domingo (doh-meen-goh)* has been ommitted from the list since you would probably never use it for the purpose of making an appointment.

[2]These phrases have been included primarily to facilitate appointment reminders made by phone. Use *del doctor* if you are calling on behalf of a *male* doctor and use *de la doctora* if you are doing so on behalf of a *female* doctor.

Practical Activities II

A) Oral Practice

1. Following the instructions given in the **NOTES** section, create your calendar overlay cards and the sheet described for negotiating appointment times. In pairs, take turns practicing making appointments with neither partner speaking ANY ENGLISH at all. Treat this as an interoffice encounter where the person making the appointment can interact directly with the patient.

2. Working in pairs, turn your desks/chairs so that you are back to back with your partner (this is to simulate a phone call in which the two persons interacting cannot see one another and must depend only on oral communication). Practice making appointments as if on the phone while still using your cards and time sheet. Don't forget to confirm the appointment after you have arranged it. Both partners should keep track of the appoinment times to check one another for correctness after completing the "phone call."

B) Telling time

Instructions: Draw the hands on the blank clock faces according to the SPANISH phrase given below each one. Then, label the hands with the appropriate number. Lastly, write A.M. or P.M. above each clock indicating the time of day of the appointment. Only look back at the phrases in the chapter after you have finished to check your answers.

Su cita es . . .

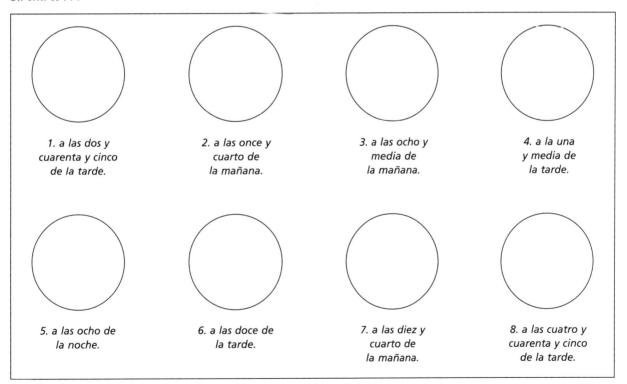

| 1. a las dos y cuarenta y cinco de la tarde. | 2. a las once y cuarto de la mañana. | 3. a las ocho y media de la mañana. | 4. a la una y media de la tarde. |

| 5. a las ocho de la noche. | 6. a las doce de la tarde. | 7. a las diez y cuarto de la mañana. | 8. a las cuatro y cuarenta y cinco de la tarde. |

Cyber-Investigation

Do an Internet search for HISPANICS and PUNCTUALITY. Then compare and contrast their concept of time and puntuality with that of our mentality in the United States. How do they differ? Why do they differ? Are there any similarities? How might the Hispanic perspective of time impact health-related issues on a broader scale?

Chapter 3

Health Care Coverage and Payment

Before You Begin

Do not be surprised by the lack of health insurance coverage . For many Hispanics, it is relative to their economic situation, and although employers may offer it as a benefit, they will refuse it since they cannot afford it or prefer not to have the money taken out of their pay. Likewise, it is less probable that they will have private or governmental health insurance though some may be covered by Medicaid. For this reason, cash will typically be the preferred means of payment.

Some confusion may arise when presenting Hispanic clients with numbers which include decimals and commas. Typically, in Spanish, numbers are written with a comma in place of a decimal and vice versa. Therefore, the sum in English of *1,250.75* would appear as *1.250,75* in Spanish.

Phrases

English	Pronunciation & Spanish
1. Do you have health insurance?	*tee^ay-nay say-**goo**-roh **may**-dee-koh?* ¿Tiene seguro médico?
2. Respond yes, no or I don't know, please.	*rray-**spohn**-dah see, noh oh noh say, pohr fah-**bohr**.* Responda sí, no o no sé, por favor.
3. Do you have a . . . card?	*tee^ay-nay lah tahr-**hay**-tah day . . .* ¿Tiene la tarjeta de . . .
Medicare?	Medicare?
Medicaid?	Medicaid?
health insurance?	*say-**goo**-roh **may**-dee-koh?* seguro médico?
Social Security?	*say-**goo**-roh soh-**see^ahl**?* seguro social?
4. Do you have a driver's license?	*tee^**ay**-nay lee-**sayn**-see^ah **pah**-rah kohn-doo-**seer**?* ¿Tiene licencia para conducir?
5. Do you have some form of (picture) I.D.?	*tee^**ay**-nay ahl-**goo**-nah **foor**-mah day ee-dayn-tee-fee-kah-**see^ohn** ¿Tiene alguna forma de identificación* *(kohn **foh**-toh)?* (con foto)?

6. May I see it?

*pway-doh **bayr**-lah?*
¿Puedo verla?

7. I need to make a copy of your

*nay-say-**see**-toh sah-**kahr koh**-pee^ah day . . .*
Necesito sacar copia de . . .

Medicare Card.

*lah tahr-**hay**-tah day Medicare.*
la tarjeta de Medicare.

Medicaid Card.

*lah tarh-**hay**-tah day Medicaid.*
la tarjeta de Medicaid.

health insurance card.

*lah tarh-**hay**-tah day say-**goo**-roh **may**-dee-koh.*
a tarjeta de seguro médico.

Social Security Card.

*lah tarh-**hay**-tah day say-**goo**-roh soh-**see**^ahl.*
la tarjeta de seguro social.

driver's license.

*soo lee-**sayn**-see^ah **pah**-rah kohn-doo-**seer**.*
su licencia para conducir.

I.D.

*soo ee-dayn-tee-fee-kah-**see**^ohn.*
su identificación.

8. Who will pay the account?

*kee^ayn pah-gah-**rah** lah **kwayn**-tah?*
¿Quién pagará la cuenta?

9. I will.

*yoh (**mees**-moh/mah).*
Yo (mismo/a).[1]

10. You need to pay . . .

*nay-say-**see**-tah pah-**gahr** lah . . .*
Necesita pagar la . . .

half

*mee-**tahd***
mitad

a third

*tayr-**sayr**-ah **pahr**-tay*
tercera parte

a fourth

*kwahr**-tah **pahr**-tay*
cuarta parte

today / up front.

*oyl day ahn-tay-**mah**-noh.*
hoy/ de antemano.

11. Full payment is preferred at

*ays pray-fay-**ree**-blay ayl **pah**-goh ayn-**tay**-roh*
Es preferible el pago entero

the time of service.

*ah lah **oh**-rah day sayr-**bee**-see^ohs rrayn-**dee**-dohs.*
a la hora de servicios rendidos.

12. Would you like to pay . . .

*kee-**see**^ay-rah pah-**gahr** . . .*
¿Quisiera pagar . . .

in cash?

*ayn ay-fayk-**tee**-boh?*
en efectivo?

with a credit / debit card?

*kohn tahr-**hay**-tah day **kray**-dee-toh / **day**-bee-toh?*
con tarjeta de crédito / débito?

with a personal check?	*kohn oon **chay**-kay payr-soh-**nahl**?* con un cheque personal?
13. We don't accept . . .	*noh ah-sayp-**tah**-mohs . . .* No aceptamos . . .
personal checks.	***chay**-kays payr-soh-**nah**-lays.* cheques personales.
this credit card.	***ay**-stah tahr-**hay**-tah day **kray**-dee-toh.* esta tarjeta de crédito.
14. How much can you pay (today)?	***kwahn**-toh **pway**-day pah-**gahr** (oy)?* ¿Cuánto puede pagar (hoy)?
15. We can set up a payment plan.	*poh-**day**-mohs ah-rray-**glahr** oon plahn day **pah**-goh.* Podemos arreglar un plan de pago.[2]
16. We can submit your claim to	*poh-**day**-mohs soh-may-**tayr** soo* Podemos someter su
your medical insurance provider.	*rray-klah-mah-**see^ohn** ah soo proh-bay-ay-**door** day say-**goo**-roh* reclamación a su proveedor de seguro
	***may**-dee-koh.* médico.
17. Your visit today will cost this.	*lah bee-**see**-tah day oy lay kohs-tah-**rah ay**-stoh.* La visita de hoy le costará esto.[3]

Notes

[1] This phrase literally means "I myself," though you may just hear "Yo." With "mismo/a" it is more emphatic. A male would use *mismo* and a female would use *misma*.

[2] When setting up a payment plan, use the calendar overlays from Chapter 2 to negotiate payment dates and the necessary phrases from this section to decide on the payment amount.

[3] Write the cost on paper and point to it as you say this phrase.

Practical Activities

A) Oral Practice

Instructions: Using SPANISH only, communicate the following to a partner as if (s)he were a Hispanic client/patient.

1. Ask if the client/patient has some form of I.D., ask to see it, then request to make a photocopy.
2. Let the client/patient know that a third of the payment is due up front and ask how the patient/client would like to pay. Tell the client/patient you do not accept personal checks.
3. Show the client/patient on a sheet of paper how much the visit today will cost. Ask for a fourth of the payment today and then explain you can set up a payment plan.

B) Word Association

Instructions: Without looking back in the chapter, identify the SPANISH vocabulary from this chapter given below as *a (a form of I. D.)*, *b (a form of health care coverage)*, *c (a method of payment)* or *d (a required payment amount)* by writing the corresponding letter in the blank provided. Check your answers after you have finished.

1. ___ pago entero

2. ___ licencia para conducir

3. ___ cheque personal

4. ___ mitad

5. ___ tarjeta de crédito

6. ___ efectivo

7. ___ identificación con foto

8. ___ plan de pago

9. ___ tarjeta de seguro médico

10. ___ tarjeta de seguro social

C) Short Answer Questions

Instructions: Answer the following questions based on information you learned in this chapter.

1. According to the **Before You Begin** section, what is the significant difference between numbers written in English and those written in Spanish?

2. Find two or three examples of this either on the Internet, or in a Spanish only or bilingual periodical or flyer.

Cyber-Investigation

What percentage of Hispanics do carry some sort of health insurance? Are there demographic breakdowns to this information? Aside from the few factors mentioned in the **Before You Begin** section, what are some other reasons why Hispanics would be less likely to have some sort of health care coverage?

_____

_____

_____

_____

_____

_____

_____

_____

_____

_____

_____

_____

_____

_____

_____

_____

_____

_____

Chapter 4

Obtaining Patient Information

Before You Begin

The date in Spanish is reversed from the date in English. In Spanish, you always begin with the day rather than with the month. Always clarify or ask for clarification of dates using a calendar if you are unsure. You may choose to use a calendar as a visual reference to make sure there is no miscommunication. Here are a few examples:

Spanish: The 25th of March of 2006 = 25/3/2006

English: March 25th, 2006 = 3/25/2006

Spanish: The 1st of April of 2006 = 1/4/2006

English: April 1st, 2006 = 4/1/2006

For most medical professionals, the personal information provided by a patient is considered to be accurate and truthful. However, this same patient information may not be the most reliable source for the identification of some Hispanic patients. Many undocumented Hispanics who are illegally employed may be doing so under an alias or assumed name. In addition, they may be using fraudulent documents to gain and maintain employment. The fear associated with being discovered using a false identity often disuades them from seeking out the necessary medical attention or forces them to wait until a situation becomes dire.

Phrases

English	Pronunciation & Spanish
1. I need to ask you some questions, please.	*nay-say-**see**-toh ah-**sayr**-lay **oo**-nahs pray-**goon**-tahs pohr fah-**bohr**.* Necesito hacerle unas preguntas, por favor.
2. What is your full name?	*kwahl ays soo **nohm**-bray kohm-**play**-toh?* ¿Cuál es su nombre completo?
3. When were you born?	***kwahn**-doh nah-**see^oh**?* ¿Cuándo nació?[1]
4. Are you married?	*ay-**stah** kah-**sah**-doh/dah?* ¿Está casado/a?[2]
5. Are you divorced?	*ay-**stah** dee-boor-**see^ah**-doh/dah?* ¿Está divorciado/a?[2]
6. Are you single?	*ays sohl-**tay**-roh/rah?* ¿Es soltero/a?[2]

7. Are you widowed?	*ays **bee^oo**-doh/dah?* ¿Es viudo/a?[2]
8. What is your husband's/wife's name?	***kohm**-moh say **yah**-mah soo ay-**spoh**-soh/sah?* ¿Cómo se llama su esposo/a?[2]
9. What is the child's name?	***kohm**-moh say **yah**-mah ayl **nee**-nyoh / lah **nee**-nyah?* ¿Cómo se llama el niño / la niña?[3]
10. Is the child your dependent?	*ays ayl **nee**-nyoh / lah **nee**-nyah soo day-payn-**dee^ayn**-tay?* ¿Es el niño / la niña su dependiente?[3]
11. What is your address?	*kwahl ays soo dee-rayk-**see^ohn**?* ¿Cuál es su dirección?[1]
12. What is your phone number?	*kwahl ays soo **noo**-may-roh day tay-**lay**-foh-noh?* ¿Cuál es su número de teléfono?[1]
13. Do you work?	*trah-**bah**-hah?* ¿Trabaja?
14. How long have you worked there?	*pohr **kwahn**-toh **tee^aym**-poh ah trah-bah-**hah**-doh ah-**yee**?* ¿Por cuánto tiempo ha trabajado allí?[1]
15. What is your work address?	*kwahl ays lah dee-rayk-**see^ohn** day soo trah-**bah**-hoh?* ¿Cuál es la dirección de su trabajo?[1]
16. What is the phone number of your workplace?	*kwahl ays ayl **noo**-may-roh day tay-**lay**-foh-noh* ¿Cuál es el número de teléfono *day soo trah-**bah**-hoh?* de su trabajo?[1]
17. Can we call you at work?	*poh-**day**-mohs yah-**mahr**-lay ayn ayl trah-**bah**-hoh?* ¿Podemos llamarle en el trabajo?
18. Does you husband/wife work?	*trah-**bah**-hah soo ay-spoh-soh/sah?* ¿Trabaja su esposo/a?[2]
19. How long has (s)he worked there?	*pohr **kwahn**-toh **tee^aym**-poh ah trah-bah-hah-doh ah-**yee**?* ¿Por cuánto tiempo ha trabajado allí?[4]
20. What is his/her work address?	*kwahl ays lah dee-rayk-**see^ohn** day soo trah-**bah**-hoh?* ¿Cuál es la dirección de su trabajo?[4]
21. What is the phone number of his/her workplace?	*kwahl ays ayl **noo**-may-roh day tay-**lay**-foh-noh* ¿Cuál es el número de teléfono *day soo trah-**bah**-hoh?* de su trabajo?[4]
22. Can we call him/her at work?	*poh-**day**-mohs yah-**mahr**-lay ayn ayl trah-**bah**-hoh?* ¿Podemos llamarle en el trabajo?[4]

Notes

[1] If possible, have the patient write this information for you. When obtaining the duration of employment use *days* from the additional vocabulary words at the end of this section. The singular and plural forms are indicated.

² These questions have two forms. For example, *¿Está casado?* is used when addressing a male and *¿Está casada?* is used when addressing a female. This is true for any of the questions you see that give you these two options: *casado/a*. Just remember, *-o* for males and *-a* for females.

³ These two questions have been included in the case that the parent or guardian is bringing in a child for an appointment. Chances are you would still conduct the conversation with the parent/guardian, although you need to know these pieces of information about the child. To avoid confusion, when you arrive to these two questions during your conversation with the parent/guardian, point to the child. When you have passed these two questions, reacknowledge the parent/guardian (a simple hand gesture toward the person will work) so there is no misunderstanding of the answers required for the questions that will follow.

⁴ Though these questions are the same as those asked directly to the client in the *you* form, they will make sense in context only after you have asked the questions *Does your husband/wife work?* Also, remember to have the client write the answers for you.

Additional Vocabulary

English	Pronunciation & Spanish
1. day(s)	*dee-ah(s)* día(s)
2. month(s)	*mays (**may**-says)* mes (meses)
3. week(s)	*say-**mah**-nah(s)* semana(s)
4. year(s)	***ah**-nyoh(s)* año(s)

Practical Activities

A) Oral Practice

Instructions: Using only SPANISH, prepare a conversation with a male and female classmate in which you obtain the patient information indicated. Make sure to use the correct gender-specific phrases when needed. Patient responses may be fictitious.

1. Obtain the following information from a female patient - name, date of birth, marital status, work phone number and duration of employment.
2. Obtain the following information from a male patient - state you will ask him some questions, then ask for name, marital status, wife's name, if she works (answer will be *sí*), where, her work phone and can she be called at work.

B) Matching

Instructions: Match the SPANISH phrase with the answer it would elicit from a Spanish speaker. Be careful to pay attention to phrases referring to *males* and *females*. Remember, in most cases they would be writing the information for you.

1. ___ ¿Cuándo nació?	a. No, divorciado.
2. ___ ¿Por cuánto tiempo ha trabajado allí?	b. Sí, está bien.
3. ___ ¿Cómo se llama su esposa?	c. 1234 Harris Drive.
4. ___ ¿Cuál es su número de teléfono?	d. Pedro Saavedra Gomez.
5. ___ ¿Está casada?	e. 14/01/1983.
6. ___ ¿Es soltero?	f. Juana Carolina.
7. ___ ¿Cuál es la dirección de su trabajo?	g. No, soltera.
8. ___ ¿Podemos llamarle en el trabajo?	h. 6 meses (months).
9. ___ ¿Cómo se llama su niño?	i. 919-555-1635.
10. ___ ¿Cuál es su nombre completo, señor?	j. Carlos.

C) Brief Response

Instructions: Provide the appropriate responses for the following items.

1. Give examples from this chapter of phrases that would apply only to *males*.

2.   Give examples from this chapter of phrases that would apply only to *females*.

3.   What are the notable differences between the phrases for *males* and *females?*

Cyber-Investigation

What might be some reasons why a Hispanic patient would be reluctant to share his or her patient information or that of a child or family member? Try to find sources that support your opinions.

Chapter 5

Medical History

Section 1
Personal Medical History

Before You Begin

Many Hispanics will readily agree with things you may say as a medical professional even though the contrary may be true. You may want to interject from time to time with the question "*¿Comprende qué es —?*" *(Do you understand what—is?)* in order to get an idea of the patient's true level of comprehension, since many times medications, illnesses, conditions, etc. may be known by more popular terminology. Even though you may not be able to offer an alternative name or phrase, you will at least not be recording erroneous medical information.

Two very important health issues that affect Hispanics are cirrhosis and alcoholism. Also, the use of narcotics account for a disproportionate number of deaths among Hispanics.

Phrases

English	Pronunciation & Spanish
1. How old are you?	*kwahn-tohs **ah**-nyohs **tee^ay**-nay?* ¿Cuántos años tiene?[1]
2. When did you have your last physical?	*kwahn-doh **too**-boh soo **ool**-tee-moh ayk-**sah**-mayn **may**-dee-koh?* ¿Cuándo tuvo su último examen médico?[1]
3. Are you pregnant?	*ay-**stah** aym-bah-rah-**sah**-dah?* ¿Está embarazada?
4. Do you understand what — is?	*kohm-**prayn**-day kay ays —-?* ¿Comprende qué es —-?
5. Are you allergic to . . .	*tee^**ay**-nay ah-**layr**-hee^ahs ah . . .* ¿Tiene alergias a . . .
aspirin?	*ah-spee-**ree**-nah?* aspirina?
Demerol?	*day-may-**rohl**?* Demerol?
iodine?	*ee^**oh**-doh?* iodo?
morphine?	*moor-**fee**-nah?* morfina?

31

penicillin?	*pay-nee-see-**lee**-nah?* penicilina?
sulfa?	***sool**-fah?* sulfa?
Valium?	***bah**-lee^oom* Valium?
anesthetics?	*lah ah-nay-**stay**-see^ah?* la anestesia?
other drugs?	***oh**-trahs **droh**-gahs?* otras drogas?[1]

6. Do you suffer or have you suffered	***soo**-fray oh ah soo-**free**-doh day . . .* ¿Sufre o ha sufrido
from...	*day . . .* de . . . [2]
anemia?	*ah-**nay**-mee^ah?* anemia?
arthritis?	*ahr-**tree**-tees?* artritis?
asthma?	***ahs**-mah?* asma?
cancer?	***cahn**-sayr?* cáncer?
anxiety?	*ahn-see^ay-**dahd**?* ansiedad?
depression?	*day-pray-**see^ohn**?* depresión?
sinusitis?	*see-noo-**see**-tees?* sinusitis?
bulimia?	*boo-**lee**-mee^ah?* bulimia?
anorexia?	*ah-noh-**rayk**-see^ah?* anorexia?
paralysis?	*pah-**rah**-lee-sees?* parálisis?
hemmorhoids?	*ay-moh-**rroy**-days?* hemorroides?
persistent cough	*tohs payr-see-**stayn**-tay?* tos persistente?
lactose intolerance?	*een-toh-lay-**rayn**-see^ah **lahk**-tay^ah?* intolerencia láctea?

venereal diseases/STDs?	*ayn-fayr-may-**dah**-days bay-**nay**-ray^ahs?* enfermedades venéreas?	
hypertension/high blood pressure?	*ee-payr-tayn-**see**^ohn?* hipertensión?	
hypotension/low blood pressure?	*ee-poh-tayn-**see**^ohn?* hipotensión?	
heart problems?	*proh-**blay**-mahs kahr-**dee**-ah-cohs?* problemas cardíacos?	
circulatory problems?	*proh-**blay**-mahs seer-koo-lah-**toh**-ree^ohs?* problemas circulatorios?	
nervous problems?	*proh-**blay**-mahs nayr-**bee**^oh-sohs?* problemas nerviosos?	
other medical problems?	***oh**-trohs proh-**blay**-mahs **may**-dee-kohs?* otros problemas médicos?	

7. Do you suffer from . . .	***soo**-fray day . . .* Sufre de . . .
diabetes?	*dee^ah-**bay**-tays?* diabetes?
hyperglycemia?	*ee-payr-glee-**say**-mee^ah?* hiperglicemia?
hepatitis?	*ay-pah-**tee**-tees?* hepatitis?
herpes?	***ayr**-pays?* herpes?
HIV	*bay-ee-**ah**-chay?* VIH?
AIDS?	***see**-dah?* SIDA?
any other illness?	***oh**-trah ayn-fayr-may-**dahd**?* otra enfermedad?

8. Have you ever suffered a . . .	*ah soo-**free**-doh . . .* ¿Ha sufrido . . .
stroke?	*day-**rrah**-may say-ray-**brahl**?* derrame cerebral?
heart attack?	*ah-**tah**-kay kahr-**dee**-ah-koh?* ataque cardíaco?

9. Have you ever had surgery?	*ah tay-**nee**-doh see-roo-**hee**-ah?* ¿Ha tenido cirugía?

	fway . . .
10. Was it . . .	¿Fue . . .
	*ah-payn-dayk-toh-**mee**-ah?*
an appendectomy?	apendectomía?
	*ee-stay-rayk-toh-**mee**-ah?*
a hysterectomy?	histerectomía?
	*day **say**-noh?*
breast surgery?	de seno?
	*day koh-rah-**sohn**?*
heart surgery?	de corazón?
	*day **koh**-lohn?*
colon surgery?	de colon?
	*day **oo**-tay-roh?*
uterine surgery?	de útero?
	*day oh-**bah**-ree^oh?*
ovarian surgery?	de ovario?
	*day rree-**nyohn**?*
kidney surgery?	de riñon?
	*day **ee**-gah-doh?*
liver surgery?	de hígado?
	*day ay-**stoh**-mah-goh?*
stomach surgery?	de estómago?
	*day **proh**-stah-tah?*
prostate surgery?	de próstata?
	*day ah-**meeg**-dah-lahs?*
a tonsillectomy?	de amígdalas?
	*day tee-**roy**-days?*
a thyroidectomy?	de tiroides?
	*day **kee**-stay oh-**bah**-ree-koh?*
for an ovarian cyst?	de quiste ovárico?
	*day **kahl**-koo-lohs rray-**nah**-lays?*
for kidney stones?	de cálculos renales?[3]
	***pah**-rah ay-moh-**rroy**-days?*
for hemorrhoids?	para hemorroides?
	*day **ayr**-nee^ah?*
for a hernia?	de hernia?
	***oh**-troh **tee**-poh day see-roo-**hee**-ah?*
another type of surgery?	otro tipo de cirugía?[1]

	***oo**-sah **droh**-gahs?*
11. Do you use drugs?	¿Usa drogas?

12. Have you ever used drugs?	*ah oo-**sah**-doh **droh**-gahs?* ¿Ha usado drogas?
13. Have you ever been treated for a	*ah **see**-doh trah-**tah**-doh/dah pohr oon* ¿Ha sido tratado/a por un
drug problem?	*proh-**blay**-mah day **droh**-gahs?* problema de drogas?
14. Do you drink (alcohol)?	***toh**-mah ahl-koh-**ohl**?* ¿Toma alcohol?
15. How many drinks	***kwahn**-tahs bay-**bee**-dahs ahl-koh-**oh**-lee-kahs* ¿Cuántas bebidas alcohólicas
do you have in a week?	***toh**-mah pohr say-**mah**-nah?* toma por semana?[1]

Notes

[1] If possible, have the patient/client write the answers to these questions for you.

[2] For a list of more health problems, see the corresponding **APPENDIX**. Some alternate expressions have been listed.

[3] To indicate "gallstones," say *cálculos biliares (bee-lee-ah-rays)*.

Practical Activites I

A) Oral Practice

Instructions: For #1, working in pairs and using ONLY SPANISH, act out the situation according to the prompts provided. After you have finished, switch roles and act it out again, providing different phrases and expressions than those used the first time through. For #2, obtain the information indicated from the patient using ONLY SPANISH. Remember to switch roles after the first time through.

1. A nurse asks a patient: if (s)he is allergic to —- (choose 4 items from this chapter); if (s)he suffers from — (choose 3 ailments); if (s)he has ever had surgery — (choose 4 different options).
2. A doctor needs the following information from a patient: age; date of last physical; if (s)he is diabetic or hypoglycemic; has an allergy to morphine or any other drug; has had a heart attack or stroke; uses or has ever used drugs; drinks and how many times per week.

B) Cognates

Instructions: Read the explanation of a *cognate* then complete the exercise.

In Spanish, a *cognate* is a word that looks and sounds similar to the English word and has the same meaning. This makes them much easier to learn for the English speaker studying Spanish since there is instant word association. Below is a list of cognates from this chapter. Try to write the ENGLISH word for each one without having to look back in the chapter. Check your answer when you are done.

Spanish	English		Spanish	English
1. hipertensión	_____		6. próstata	_____
2. depresión	_____		7. ataque	_____
3. persistente	_____		8. sufre	_____
4. aspirina	_____		9. drogas	_____
5. apcndectomía	_____		10. alcohólicas	_____

C) Brief Response

Instructions: Provide the appropriate information for the following items.

1. Find 3–4 examples of cognates from each previous chapter.

2. Did you find any that were *exactly* like their English counterparts? If so which ones? What may be some reasons why cognates exist?

_____

_____

_____

_____

_____

Cyber-Investigation

In addition to *cirrhosis* and *alcoholism*, find a minimun of **three** other health-related problems and issues that greatly affect the Hispanic population and explain why. Were you able to anticipate your findings or were you surprised? Explain.

_____

_____

_____

_____

_____

_____

_____

_____

_____

_____

_____

_____

Section II
Family Medical History

Before You Begin

Overall, Hispanics are less comfortable talking about their family medical history and are more likely to associate shame or embarrassment with details regarding the condition of their health or the health of a family member. Likewise, Hispanics tend to be less knowledgeable of their own family medical history and health-related issues.

Diet plays a large role in obesity with Hispanics. For many of them, their main diet is high in saturated fats and many Mexican-Americans tend to have higher cholesterol and triglyceride levels than their Amercian counterparts. Likewise, economically disadvantaged Hispanics are at greater risk for high blood pressure (hypertension) which often times goes undiagnosed and untreated.

Phrases

English	Pronunciation & Spanish
1. I am going to ask you some questions	*lay boy ah ah-**sayr** oo-nahs pray-**goon**-tahs* Le voy a hacer unas preguntas
about your family medical history.	***soh**-bray soo ee-**stoh**-ree^ah **may**-dee-kah fah-mee-**lee^ahr**.* sobre su historia médica familiar.
2. Answer with ...	*kohn-**tay**-stay kohn ...* Conteste con ...
no	*noh* no
father	***pah**-dray* padre
mother	***mah**-dray* madre
brother	*ayr-**mah**-noh* hermano
sister	*ayr-**mah**-nah* hermana
and/or grandparents	*ee / oh ah-**bway**-lohs* y/o abuelos
please.	*pohr fah-**bohr**.* por favor.
3. Is there history of ...	*ah^ee ee-**stoh**-ree^ah day ...* ¿Hay historia de ...
drug use?	***oo**-soh day **droh**-gahs?* uso de drogas?

arthritis?	*ahr-**tree**-tees?* artritis?
birth defects?	*day-**fayk**-tohs day nah-see-**mee^ayn**-toh?* defectos de nacimiento?
excessive bleeding?	*sahn-**grah**-doh ayk-say-**see**-boh?* sangrado excesivo?
cancer?	***kahn**-sayr?* cáncer?
colon cancer?	***kayn**-sayr dayl **koh**-lohn?* cáncer del colon?
stomach cancer?	***kahn**-sayr **gah**-stree-koh?* cáncer gástrico?
(Age at diagnosis?)	*ay-**dahd** ahl dee^ahg-**noh**-stee-koh?* (¿Edad al diagnóstico?)
colitis?	*koh-**lee**-tees?* colitis?
colon polyps?	***poh**-lee-pohs dayl **koh**-lohn?* pólipos del colon?
Crohn's disease?	*ayn-fayr-may-**dahd** day krohn?* enfermedad de Crohn?
diabetes?	*dee^ah-**bay**-tays?* diabetes?
heart problems?	*proh-**blay**-mahs kahr-**dee**-ah-kohs?* problemas cardíacos?
high blood pressure?	*ee-payr-tayn-**see^ohn**?* hipertensión?
liver disease?	*ayn-fayr-may-**dahd** dayl **ee**-gah-doh?* enfermedad del hígado?
lung diseases?	*ayn-fayr-may-**dah**-days pool-moh-**nah**-rays?* enfermedades pulmonares?
thrombosis or stroke/cerebral embolism?	*trohm-**boh**-sees oh aym-boh-**lees**-moh say-ray-**brahl**?* trombosis o embolismo cerebral?
blood clots?	*koh-**ah**-goo-lohs sahn-**ghee**-nay-ohs?* coágulos sanguíneos?
tuberculosis?	*too-bayr-koo-**loh**-sees?* tuberculosis?
thyroid disease?	*ayn-fayr-may-**dahd** tee-**roy**-day^ah?* enfermedad tiroidea?
ulcer?	***ool**-say-rah?* úlcera?

other health problems?	*oh-trohs proh-**blay**-mahs day sah-**lood**?* otros problemas de salud?[1]
4. For these questions, respond	*pah-rah **ay**-stahs pray-**goon**-tahs* Para estas preguntas,
yes, no, or I don't know.	*rray-**spohn**-day see noh oh noh say.* responde sí, no, o no sé.
5. Is your ... alive?	*ay-**stah bee**-boh soo ...* ¿Está vivo su . . .
father	***pah**-dray?* padre?
brother	*ayr-**mah**-noh?* hermano?
grandfather	*ah-**bway**-loh?* abuelo?
6. Is your ... healthy?	*ay-**stah sah**-noh soo ...* ¿Está sano su ...
father	***pah**-dray?* padre?
brother	*ayr-**mah**-noh?* hermano?
grandfather	*ah-**bway**-loh?* abuelo?
7. Is your ... alive?	*ay-**stah bee**-bah soo ...* ¿Está viva su ...
mother	***mah**-dray?* madre?
sister	*ayr-**mah**-nah?* hermana?
grandmother	*ah-**bway**-lah?* abuela?
8. Is your ... healthy?	*ay-**stah sah**-nah soo ...* ¿Está sana su ...
mother	***mah**-dray?* madre?
sister	*ayr-**mah**-nah?* hermana?
grandmother	*ah-**bway**-lah?* abuela?
9. Do you use tobacco products?	*oo-sah tah-**bah**-koh?* Usa tabaco?

10.	Have you ever used tobacco products?	*ah oo-**sah**-doh tah-**bah**-koh?* ¿Ha usado tabaco?
11.	Do you smoke?	***foo**-mah?* ¿Fuma?
12.	Have you ever smoked?	*ah foo-**mah**-doh?* ¿Ha fumado?

Notes

[1] If possible, have the patient write these answers down for you.

Practical Activities II

A) Oral Practice

Instructions: Before beginning, each student should *invent* an identity in which (s)he also has an *invented* family medical history. This will allow for answers to vary without feeling as though you are sharing *true* confidential information with others. In doing so, go through the phrases in this chapter and quickly decide what your responses will be. Jot them down on a scrap sheet of paper to use as your prompts or lightly notate your responses in pencil in your text for the sake of time. After taking the time to do this, find and a partner and follow the guidelines for the situation that follows, acting out the situation in SPANISH only. After completing the situation once, switch roles and repeat.

1. Nurse — Inform patient that (s)he will be asked questions related to family medical history. Explain how to respond to the questions. Ask five questions from set 3 (expressions from section number 3 of this chapter). Explain how to answer yes/no questions. Then ask about male then female relatives. Ask about tobacco use. If at anytime you do not understand, ask the patient to please repeat.

Follow-up:

As you question the patient about his/her medical history, note his/her responses. Ask your partner to then check what you wrote against the notes (s)he made regarding the *invented* family medical history to verify your comprehension.

B) ¿Hombre o mujer? (Man or woman?)

Instructions: Find the words for the *male* members of the family in this chapter and those for the *female* family members. Then answer the questions.

1. How are they alike? Different?
2. Can learning one set make it easier to learn the other set? How?

C) If … then … statements

Instructions: Based on what you learned in **B) ¿Hombre o mujer?** *(Man or woman?)*, Fill in the blank with the meaning of each word according to the clues provided in the *If … then …* statements. Some you have had in this chapter and some are new. Try to complete the chart without referring to the chapter for help or asking your instructor.

1. *If* abuelo = grandfather, *then* abuela = _____.

2. *If* hermana = sister *then* hermano = _____.

3. *If* madre = mother *then* padre = _____.

4. *If* tío (**tee**-oh) = uncle *then* tía (**tee**-ah) = _____.

5. *If* prima (**pree**-mah) = (female) cousin *then* primo (**pree**-moh) = _____.

6. *If* sobrino (soh-**bree**-noh) = nephew *then* sobrina (soh-**bree**-nah) = _____.

7. *If* enfermera = (female) nurse *then* enfermero = _____.

8. *If* médico = (male) doctor *then* médica = _____.

Cyber-Investigation

In **Before You Begin** you were told that Hispanics are less likely to know their family medical history and may feel shameful of it as well. What are some of the reasons for this? Might Hispanic females be less likely to share such information than Hispanic males? Why or why not?

_____

_____

_____

_____

_____

_____

_____

_____

_____

_____

_____

_____

_____

_____

_____

_____

_____

_____

Chapter 6

Handling Office Traffic

Before You Begin

Hispanic families are very close-knit. Therefore, it would not be uncommon that more than one family member accompany a sick relative to a doctor's appointment. Likewise, since nonverbal communication is strongly influenced by respect, direct eye contact may be avoided between Hispanics and authority figures, such as medical professionals, due to a perceived class distinction. However, a family member may show respect for a medical professional by standing when he or she enters the room. Also, it would be disrespectful for the medical professional to address an elderly Hispanic person by his or her first name.

Do not forget that when speaking with a Hispanic patient you are also addressing directly or indirectly that patient's entire family. Most important decisions will be made taking into account the opinions and comments of all family members, including discussions regarding a patient's diagnosis and treatment plans.

Phrases

English	Pronunciation & Spanish
1. You may sit in the waiting room.	*pway-day sayn-tahr-say ayn lah sah-lah day ay-spay-rah.* Puede sentarse en la sala de espera.
2. You'll be called as soon as possible.	*lay yah-mahn tahn prohn-toh koh-moh poh-see-blay.* Le llaman tan pronto como posible.
3. The restrooms are over there.	*lohs sayr-bee-see^ohs ay-stahn pohr ah-yee.* Los servicios están por allí.[1]
4. Cell phones are not allowed in the doctor's office.	*noh say payr-mee-tayn lohs say-loo-lah-rays* No se permiten los celulares *ayn lah kohn-sool-tah.* en la consulta.
5. Smoking is not allowed.	*noh say foo-mah.* No se fuma.
6. Only one family member may accompany you.	*soh-loh oon mee^aym-broh fah-mee-lee^ahr* Sólo un miembro familiar *pway-day ah-kohm-pah-nyahr-lay.* puede acompañarle.
7. Come with me, please.	*pah-say pohr fah-bohr.* Pase, por favor.[1]

8. Will you follow me, please?	*may **see**-gay pohr fah-**bohr**.* ¿Me sigue, por favor?[1]
9. Wait in here, please.	*ay-**spay**-ray ah-**kee** pohr fah-**bohr**.* Espere aquí, por favor.[1]
10. The doctor will be in soon.	*ayl dohk-**tohr** bee^ay-nay **prohn**-toh.* El doctor viene pronto.[2]
11. The nurse will be in soon.	*ayl ayn-fayr-**may**-roh **bee^ay**-nay **prohn**-toh.* El enfermero viene pronto.[2]
12. Please calm your children.	*fah-**bohr** day kahl-**mahr** ah lohs **nee**-nyohs.* Favor de calmar a los niños.
13. The water fountain is over there.	*ah^ee **oo**-nah **fwayn**-tay day **ah**-gwah pohr ah-**yee**.* Hay una fuente de agua por allí.[1]
14. Please hold it down.	***kahl**-mayn-say pohr fah-**bohr**.* Cálmense, por favor.

Notes

[1] Use hand gestures to assist you in communicating these phrases. Many times, gestures/body language can aid greatly in bridging the communication gap between speakers of different languages. Also, an alternate word for *servicios* is *baños* (**bah**-*nyohs*).

[2] Though not listed, if you know the doctor or nurse to be female, use the respective gender-specific words found in previous chapters.

Practical Activities

A) Oral Response

Instructions: How would you respond, in SPANISH, to the following scenarios? Prepare your responses and present them to a classmate or small group. Do this without revealing which of the scenarios you are recreating and have your partner or group members guess which number it is below based on what they understand. After you have presented, allow your partner or other group members to do the same.

1. A patient signs in and continues to stand at the counter.
2. Three people get up to go back with a patient who has been called.
3. A patient needs to follow you to the lab and stay there until the nurse comes.
4. A parent has left some older children alone in the waiting room who are being loud.
5. An elderly man comes in smoking then asks for the restrooms.
6. A lady is talking loudly on her cell phone while her children are bothering others.

B) Brief Response

Instructions: Provide the requested information for the items below.

1. List the gender-specific words you would need to recall from previous chapters to correctly reference male and female doctors and nurses.

2. Share examples of gestures/body language with other class participants that could be used to help facilitate communication of the respective phrases in this chapter. Demonstrate them in small groups or for the class.

Cyber-Investigation

As you learned in the **Before You Begin** section, the Hispanic family is very close. What roles would the family play in the care of a sick or incapacitated family member? How do these roles differ from that of the typical American family? What would you as a medical professional need to understand in order to better serve your Hispanic patients and their family?

Chapter 7

Intake Procedures

Before You Begin

In Spanish, the word *droga* (**droh**-*gah*) does not refer to *medicine* (*medicina* pronounced *may-day-see-nah*) but rather refers to narcotics and illegal drugs. Also, the word *drogaría* (*droh-gah-**ree**-ah*) is a *false cognate* — it looks like an English word but does not mean what one may think. Instead of being a place to buy *drugs*, which is a cognate for the word *pharmacy* (*farmacia* pronounced *fahr-**mah**-see^ah*), it is store that sells all other types of products, from shampoo and soap to cleaning products. Only a *farmacia* would sell *medicina*.

Phrases

English	Pronunciation & Spanish
1. My name is —.	*may **yah**-moh —.* Me llamo —.
2. I'm nurse —.	*soy ayl ayn-fayr-**may**-roh —.* Soy el enfermero —.[1] *soy lah ayn-fayr-**may**-rah —.* Soy la enfermera —.[1]
3. Relax, please.	*ray-**lah**-hay-say pohr fah-**bohr**.* Relájese, por favor.
4. Don't worry.	*noh say pray-oh-**koo**-pay.* No se preocupe.
5. First, I am going to ask you some questions.	*pree-**may**-roh lay boy ah ah-**sayr*** Primero, le voy a hacer ***oo**-nahs pray-**goon**-tahs.* unas preguntas.
6. Respond yes or no, please.	*rray-**spohn**-dah see oh noh pohr fah-**bohr**.* Responda sí o no, por favor.
7. Are you currently taking . . . any medication? vitamins? herbal supplements?	*ahk-too^ahl-**mayn**-tay ay-**stah** toh-**mahn**-doh . . .* Actualmente, está tomando . . . *ahl-**goo**-nah may-dee-**see**-nah?* alguna medicina? *vee-tah-**mee**-nahs?* vitaminas? *proh-**dook**-tohs ayr-**bah**-lays?* productos herbales?

8. Will you write the name here for me?

*may ay-**skree**-bay ayl **nohm**-bray ah-**kee**?*
¿Me escribe el nombre aquí?[2]

9. Now, I need to . . .

*ah-**oh**-rah lay nay-say-**see**-toh . . .*
Ahora, le necesito . . .

    weigh you.

*pay-**sahr**.*
pesar.

    get your height.

*may-**deer**.*
medir.

    take your pulse.

*toh-**mahr** ayl **pool**-soh.*
tomar el pulso.

    take your blood pressure.

*toh-**mahr** lah pray-**see^ohn**.*
tomar la presión.

    take your temperature.

*toh-**mahr** lah taym-pay-rah-**too**-rah.*
tomar la temperatura.

10. Stand here.

*pohn-gah-say ah-**kee**.*
Póngase aquí.[3]

11. Hold still, please.

*ay-stay-say **kee^ay**-toh/tah pohr fah-**bohr**.*
Éstese quieto/a, por favor.[4]

12. Roll up your sleeve, please.

*soo-bah-say lah **mahn**-gah pohr fah-**bohr**.*
Súbase la manga, por favor.

13. May I have your arm?

*may dah ayl **brah**-soh?*
¿Me da el brazo?

14. Relax your arm.

*rray-**lah**-hay ayl **brah**-soh.*
Relaje el brazo.

15. Look at me.

***mee**-ray-may.*
Míreme.

16. Look straight ahead.

***mee**-ray day-**lahn**-tay.*
Mire delante.

17. Open your mouth.

***ah**-brah lah **boh**-kah.*
Abra la boca.

18. Put this under your tongue.

*pohn-gah **ay**-stoh day-**bah**-hoh day lah **layn**-gwah.*
Ponga esto debajo de la lengua.

19. Close your mouth.

*see^**ay**-rray lah **boh**-kah.*
Cierre la boca.

20. Keep it under your tongue

*mahn-**tayn**-gah-loh day-**bah**-hoh day lah*
Manténgalo debajo de la

    until I take it out.

***layn**-gwah **ah**-stah kay say loh **sah**-kay.*
lenguahasta que se lo saque.

21. Take this off.

***kee**-tay-say **ay**-stoh.*
Quítese esto.[5]

	pohn-gah-say **ay**-stoh.
22. Put this on.	Póngase esto.[5]

	*ayl dohk-**tohr** bee^**ay**-nay **prohn**-toh.*
23. The doctor will be in shortly.	El doctor viene pronto.[6]

Notes

[1] Use *el enfermero* if you are a male nurse and *la enfermera* if you are a female nurse.

[2] Have the patient write this down for you.

[3] Point to where you would like the person to stand.

[4] Use *quieto* if you are talking to a male patient and *quieta* if you are talking to a female patient.

[5] Point to the item or article of clothing you want the patient to remove, then hand the patient the item you would like for him/her to put on.

[6] Though not listed, if you know the doctor to be female, use the respective gender-specific word found in previous chapters.

Practical Activities

A) Oral Practice

Instructions: In groups of three or four, have two people stand and act out the situation as the third person or other pair supply the prompts according to the criteria given for each situation. Remember, the pair acting out the situation may ONLY use SPANISH. Pairs/partners switch to act out the same situation again before moving onto the next. Feel free to consult previous chapters if necessary for the third situation.

1. A doctor/nurse introduces him/herself, calms the patient and states (s)he will be asked questions and explains how to respond. Continue by asking the patient two questions about current medicines and supplements. Ask that (s)he write the names down for you.
2. A nurse introduces him/herself and calms the anxious patient. (S)he then gets the weight, height, blood pressure and temperature, instructing the patient what to do as (s)he carries out these procedures.
3. The nurse goes to the waiting room, calls the patient, greets the patient and asks him/her to follow. (S)he notices that two people are with the patient and states that only one may go back to the room. In the room, the nurse requests the patient take off his/her shirt and pants and put on a gown. (S)he then says the doctor will be in soon and leaves.

B) Brief Response

Instructions: Answer the questions and discuss your answers with the class or in small groups.

1. Are there more examples of gender-specific words in this chapter? If so, what are they and to whom are they directed?

2. What phrases in this chapter might have multiple uses (phrases that are able to be used in other contexts in a medical setting)? Give examples of when alternate uses might be appropriate.

Cyber-Investigation

In previous chapters you learned what a *cognate* is, however there are also *false cognates* of which English speakers must be very careful. One such example is given in **Before You Begin**. Here are some other common *false cognates* that you will need to know that are not what they seem. Find their true meanings and write them underneath each one. Then find the Spanish word for what you thought they meant. Have your instructor help you with their pronunciation and give you context for their use.

1. *constipación*   2. *embarazada*   3. *éxito*   4. *carpeta*   5. *chocar*

_____   _____   _____   _____   _____

6. *soportar*   7. *actual*   8. *asistir*   9. *parientes*   10. *recordar*

_____   _____   _____   _____   _____

Chapter 8

Immunizations and Wellness Testing for School Age Children

Section I
Taking Vitals/General Diagnostic Questions

Before You Begin

It is no surprise that Hispanic children face the same issues regarding access to health care as Hispanic adults. Hispanic children are twice as likely not to have any health care insurance as all other children combined. They face the same socioeconomic hardships as Hispanic adults, as well as the same cultural and language barriers. Also, Hispanic children are more likely to live in poverty.

On average, Hispanic children in the U.S. are more overweight than non-Hispanic white children. This is primarily due to dietary habits, and more than anything else, the consumption of sugar. This, of course, makes them much more likely to develop type-2 diabetes, which is quite common among the adult Hispanic population.

Regarding mental health, Hispanic youth experience more anxiety-related behavioral problems, drug use, and depression than their non-Hispanic counterparts. This has been linked with stress arising from assimilation problems, many of which are compounded by communication difficulties. The inability to communicate effectively is also the most common underlying source of psychiatric referrals given out by schools to Hispanic children. A study of high school students indicated that Hispanic teenagers also had more frequent thoughts of suicide than non-Hispanic students.

Phrases

English	Pronunciation & Spanish
1. Hello.	*oh-lah.* Hola.
2. I'm nurse —.	*soy ayl ayn-fayr-**may**-roh —.* Soy el enfermero —.[1] *soy lah ayn-fayr-**may**-rah —.* Soy la enfermera —.[1]
3. My name is —.	*may **yah**-moh —.* Me llamo —.
4. What's your name?	*koh-moh tay **yah**-mahs?* ¿Cómo te llamas?[2]

5. It's a pleasure to meet you.	*moo*-choh **goo**-stoh. Mucho gusto.	
6. Follow me, please.	**see**-gay-may pohr fah-**bohr**. Sígueme, por favor.	
7. Relax, please.	ray-**lah**-hay-tay pohr fah-**bohr**. Relájate, por favor.	
8. I need to . . .	tay nay-say-**see**-toh . . . Te necesito . . .	
weigh you.	pay-**sahr**. pesar.	
get your height	may-**deer**. medir.	
take your pulse.	toh-**mahr** ayl **pool**-soh. tomar el pulso.	
take your blood pressure.	toh-**mahr** lah pray-**see^ohn**. tomar la presión.	
take your temperature.	toh-**mahr** lah taym-pay-rah-**too**-rah. tomar la temperatura.	
9. Stand here.	**pohn**-tay ah-**kee**. Ponte aquí.[3]	
10. Hold still, please.	**ay**-stah-tay **kee^ay**-toh/tah pohr fah-**bohr**. Éstate quieto/a, por favor.[4]	
11. Roll up your sleeve, please.	**soo**-bay-tay lah **mahn**-gah pohr fah-**bohr**. Súbete la manga, por favor.	
12. Give me your arm.	**dah**-may ayl **brah**-soh. Dame el brazo.	
13. Relax your arm.	rray-**lah**-hah ayl **brah**-soh. Relaja el brazo.	
14. Look at me.	**mee**-rah-may. Mírame.	
15. Look straight ahead.	**mee**-rah day-**lahn**-tay. Mira delante.	
16. Open your mouth.	**ah**-bray lah **boh**-kah. Abre la boca.	
17. Put this under your tongue.	**pohn** ay-stoh day-**bah**-hoh day lah **layn**-gwah. Pon esto debajo de la lengua.	
18. Close your mouth.	**see^ay**-rrah lah **boh**-kah. Cierra la boca.	

19. Keep it under your tongue	*mahn-**tayn**-lo day-**bah**-hoh day lah **layn**-gwah* Mantenlo debajo de la lengua	
until I take it out.	***ah**-stah kay tay loh **sah**-kay.* hasta que te lo saque.	
20. Take this off.	***kee**-tah-tay **ay**-stoh.* Quítate esto.[5]	
21. Put this on.	***pohn**-tay **ay**-stoh.* Ponte esto.[5]	
22. Do you feel bad today?	*tay **see^ayn**-tays mahl oy?* ¿Te sientes mal hoy?	
23. I'm (very) sorry.	*loh **see^ayn**-toh (**moo**-choh).* Lo siento (mucho).	
24. Can you show me with your	*may **mway**-strahs kohn ayl **day**-doh* ¿Me muestras con el dedo	
finger where you hurt?	***dohn**-day tay **dway**-lay?* dónde te duele?	
25. I'm going to show you some little faces;	*tay boy ah moh-**strahr oo**-nahs kah-**ree**-tahs* Te voy a mostrar unas caritas;	
point out the one that feels like you do.	*ah-**poon**-tah ah lah kay say **see^ayn**-tah **koh**-moh too.* apunta a la que se sienta como tú.[6]	

Notes

[1] Use *el enfermero* if you are a male nurse and *la enfermera* if you are a female nurse.

[2] When talking to children/teenagers, an adult/professional will address them using a different form of the language, so to speak. Though the English phrases may make no distinction in formality, Spanish phrases do. It is important to remember this since an adult/professional addressing a child/teenager as a peer would seem rather comedic in tone. Don't worry about learning these structural differences, simply use the phrases designated for the appropriate situation.

[3] Point to where you would like the person to stand.

[4] Use *quieto* if you are talking to a male patient and *quieta* if you are talking to a female patient.

[5] Point to the item or article of clothing you want the patient to remove, then hand the patient the item you would like for him/her to put on.

[6] Use the *Child's Pain Scale* found in the **APPENDIX** for this section. For teen patients, use the *Pain Scale/Escala de dolor* found in the **APPENDIX** for Chapter 9.

Practical Activities I

A) Oral Practice

Instructions: Using the **Oral Practice** section from **Chapter 7**, recreate the three given situations making them age appropriate (meaning instead of talking to an adult, you are now speaking to a child or teenager). Add the *Additional Situation* as the fourth situation in the original set.

Additional Situation

Using the pain scale for Children, practice with a partner assessing the pain a child patient may be experiencing using the appropriate phrases and the chart to assist you.

B) Brief Response

Instructions: Answer the questions based on what you have learned throughout **Chapter 7** and **Chapter 8**.

1. What are the notable differences between the phrases used to speak to adults and those used to speak with children and teens?

2. Can you think of examples of this in English, however more subtle they may be?

C) Adult or child/teenager?

Instructions: Write *A* (**adult**) or *C* (**child/teenager**) in the space provided beside of each phrase, designating to whom the expression would be said. Check your answers against the phrases in **Chapter 7** and **Chapter 8** when you are done.

1. ___ Te necesito pesar.

2. ___ Póngase aquí.

3. ___ Míreme.

4. ___ Cierre la boca.

5. ___ Le necesito medir.

6. ___ ¿Me muestras con el dedo?

7. ___ Ponte aquí.

8. ___ Relaja el brazo.

9. ___ Sígueme, por favor.

10. ___ Quítese esto.

11. ___ Mírame.

12. ___ Cierra la boca.

Cyber-Investigation

Find a recent on-line article that directly addresses the health (either physical or mental) of Hispanic youth and give a brief report of its content to the class. After your summary of the article, reflect on what information you found to be the most surprising or shocking whether you were previously aware of it or not. Poll the class to see how many people were conscious of the information. As you listen to other classmates report on their articles, make sure to write down any information you may find helpful in assisting you in developing your knowledge of Hispanic youth and health for future reference as a medical professional.

Section II
Administering Immunizations/Vaccinations

Before You Begin

Hispanic children are 50% more likely to be overvaccinated than white children. This is largely due to the communication barrier between this population and their health care providers, and the lack of documentation of immunization histories or immunization registries. On the other hand, Hispanic parents are more likely to forgo vaccinations, not only due to their feeling *linguistically* isolated, but also because of their lack of understanding of the U.S. health care system, their immigration status, lack of insurance, or even their own level of education. Though many of these childhood diseases have been essentially eradicated in the U.S., there are many countries where they still pose a risk.

Phrases

English	Pronunciation & Spanish
1. Your child needs vaccinations	*soo **nee**-nyoh / **nee**-nyah nay-say-**see**-tah bah-**koo**-nahs* Su niño / niña necesita vacunas
to attend school or childcare.	***pah**-rah ah-see-**steer** ah lah ay-**skway**-lah oh lah gwahr-day-**ree**-ah.* para asistir a la escuela o la guardería.[1]
2. Vaccinations protect children	*lahs bah-**koo**-nahs proh-**tay**-hayn ah lohs **nee**-nyohs* Las vacunas protegena los niños
from dangerous infections.	*day een-fayk-**see^oh**-nays pay-lee-**groh**-sahs.* de infecciones peligrosas.
3. It is important for his/her health	*ays eem-pohr-**tahn**-tay **pah**-rah lah sah-**lood** day soo **nee**-nyoh / **nee**-nyah* Es importante para la salud de su niño / niña
and it is the law.	*ee ays lah lay^ee.* y es la ley.[1]
4. It is important that your child	*ays eem-pohr-**tahn**-tay kay soo **nee**-nyoh / **nee**-nyah* Es importante que su niño / niña
be vaccinated according to	*rray-**see**-bah lahs bah-**koo**-nahs say-**goon*** reciba las vacunas según
a specified schedule.	*oon kroh-noh-**grah**-mah.* un cronograma.[1]
5. You need to keep vaccination records	*nay-say-**see**-tah mahn-tay-**nayr** oon rray-**hee**-stroh day bah-**koo**-nahs* Necesita mantener un registro de vacunas
for each child.	***pah**-rah **kah**-dah **nee**-nyoh.* para cada niño.
6. We can give you your child's	*lay poh-**day**-mohs dahr ayl rray-**hee**-stroh* Le podemos dar el registro
vaccination records.	*day bah-**koo**-nahs day soo **nee**-nyoh / **nee**-nyah.* de vacunas de su niño / niña.[1]

7. You should know that the shots

day-bay sah-*bayr* kay lahs bah-*koo*-nahs
Debe saber que las vacunas

may have side effects.

pway-dayn tay-*nayr* ay-*fayk*-tohs say-koon-*dah*-ree^ohs.
pueden tener efectos secundarios.

8. For example, fever, rash and/or

pohr ay-*haym*-ploh *fee^ay*-bray sahl-poo-*yee*-doh ee / oh
Por ejemplo, fiebre, salpullido y / o

pain where the shot was given.

doh-*lohr* ayn ayl loo-*gahr* day lah een-yayk-*see^ohn*.
dolor en el lugar de la inyección.

9. Slight discomfort is common.

oo-nah *lay*-vay een-koh-moh-dee-*dahd* ays koh-*moon*.
Una leve incomodidad es común.

10. It is rare that vaccinations cause

ays *rrah*-roh kay lahs bah-*koo*-nahs proh-*doos*-kahn
Es raro que las vacunas produzcan

a serious side effect.

oo-nah rray-ahk-*see^ohn say*-ree^ah.
una reacción seria.

11. If you think your child is having a severe

see *kray*-ay kay soo *nee*-nyoh / *nee*-nyah ay-*stah* tayn-*nee^ayn*-doh *oo*-nah
Si cree que su niño / niña está teniendo una

reaction to the vaccination, call us.

rray-ahk-*see^ohn say*-ree^ah ah lah bah-*koo*-nah *yah*-may-nohs.
reacción seria a la vacuna, llámenos.[1]

12. I need to vaccinate him/her for

nay-say-*see*-toh poh-*nayr*-lay lah bah-*koo*-nah *pah*-rah . . .
Necesito ponerle la vacuna para . . .

hepatitis B.

ay-pah-*tee*-tees bay.
hepatitis B.

diphtheria.

deef-*tay*-ree^ah.
difteria.

tetanus.

tay-tah-noh.
tétano.

pertussis.

payr-*too*-sees (tohs fay-*ree*-nah).
pertusis (tos ferina).

measles.

sah-rahm-*pee^ohn*.
sarampión.

mumps.

pah-*pay*-rahs.
paperas.

rubella.

rroo-*bay*-oh-lah.
rubéola.

pneumococcal.

nay^oo-moh-*koh*-see^ah.
neumococia.

influenza.

een-*floo^ayn*-sah.
influenza.

hepatitis A.

ay-pah-*tee*-tees ah.
hepatitis A.

polio.	*poh-lee-^oh.* polio.
type B influenza.	*een-**floo-^ayn**-sah **tee**-poh bay.* influenza tipo B.
tuberculosis.	*too-bayr-koo-**loh**-sees.* tuberculosis.
chicken pox.	*bah-ree-**say**-lah.* varicela.
13. Will you help keep your child calm?	*may **pway**-day ah-yoo-**dahr** ah kahl-**mahr** ah soo **nee**-nyoh / **nee**-nyah?* ¿Me puede ayudar a calmar a su niño / niña?[1]
14. Don't worry.	*noh tay pray-oh-**koo**-pays.* No te preocupes.[2]
15. Don't cry.	*noh **yoh**-rays.* No llores.[2]
16. It will be very quick.	*bah ah sayr mwee **rrah**-pee-doh.* Va a ser muy rápido.[2]
17. Hold still, please.	***ay**-stah-tay **kee-^ay**-toh/tah pohr fah-**bohr**.* Estate quieto / a,[3] por favor.[2]
18. This won't hurt.	*noh tay bah ah doh-**layr**.* No te va a doler.[2]
19. We're done.	*tayr-mee-**nah**-mohs.* Terminamos.
20. Your child needs to return	*soo **nee**-nyoh / **nee**-nyah nay-say-**see**-tah bohl-**bayr*** Su niño / niña necesita volver
on or after his/her . . .	*ayn oh day-**spways** day soo . . .* en o después de su . . .[1]
first	*pree-**mayr*** primer
second	*say-**goon**-doh* segundo
third	*tayr-**sayr*** tercer
fourth	***kwahr**-toh* cuarto
fifth	***keen**-toh* quinto
sixth	***sayk**-stoh* sexto

seventh	*sayp-tee-moh* séptimo
eighth	*ohk-tah-boh* octavo
ninth	*noh-bay-noh* noveno
tenth	*day-see-moh* décimo
birthday for the next dose.	*koom-play-ah-nyohs pah-rah lah prohk-see-mah doh-sees.* cumpleaños para la próxima dosis.[4]

Notes

[1] Use *niño* with a *male child* and *niña* with a *female child*.

[2] These phrases have been included for when you are directly addressing the child during the vaccinations. Therefore, they have been written to reflect communication between an adult and a child. Use them freely for comforting and calming. Remember, your delivery will have much to do with the way they are perceived.

[3] Use *quieto* with a *male child* and *quieta* with a *female child*.

[4] After *décimo (tenth)* Spanish uses cardinal numbers instead of ordinal numbers. See Chapter 18 for cardinal numbers and their pronunciation.

Practical Activities II

A) Oral Practice

Introduction: In groups of two or three (possible roles may include *nurse, doctor, parent, child, etc.*), act out the following situations according to the information you are asked to provide. Recreate each situation until each person or group member has had the opportunity to play each role.

1. Nurse explains to parent (and child) the importance of vaccinations and why they are necessary and what the risks are of not being vaccinated.
2. Nurse explains to parent (and child) what can be expected after being vaccinated, what to do should a reaction occur and the need for shot records.
3. Nurse tells the parent (and child) what shots are going to be administered (3-4 examples). Meanwhile, the child becomes nervous and rowdy. The nurse asks for help to calm the child and then tries soothing the child with appropriate expressions (hint: watch your tone since you are working with a child and not an adult).

B) Cronograma de Vacunas (Vaccination Schedule)

Instructions: Translate the following *cronograma de vacunas* from Spanish to English. Remember to look for *cognates* that will help you translate the information as well as words and expressions you have had in this chapter.

Vacunas necesarias para asistir a la escuela o la guardería:*

grados ➤ vacunas ▼	kinder	grados 1–5	grado 6	grados 6–9	grados 10–12
varicela	1 dosis en o depués del primer cumpleaños	no requerida	verificación de vacuna requerida	no requerida	no requerida
difteria, tétanos, pertusis (acelular)	4 dosis con la última dosis en o despúes del cuarto cumpleaños	pertusis no es requerida depués del séptimo cumpleaños	verificación de vacunas requerida		
polio	3 dosis con la última dosis en o después del cuarto cumpleaños				
sarampión, paperas, rubéola	2 dosis en o depués del primer cumpleaños seperadas por 28 días				
hepatitis B	3 dosis			no requerida	

* This chart is for the purpose of practice only and is not intended to be used as a schedule for actual vaccination administration.

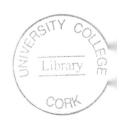

C) Brief Response

Instructions: Provide the requested answer for each set of questions.

1. How do you refer to a *male* child? A *female* child?

2. When making these distinctions, what changes do you notice in the structure of the phrases? (meaning - How do the phrases appear different?)

3. The tone in which you speak certain phrases can also impact the effectiveness of your communication. Practice calming a child using the appropriate phrases given in this chapter. How might you change your delivery when speaking to a shy, quiet child opposed to a loud, rambunctious one? How might you respectfully employ the assistance of the parent or accompanying adult?

Cyber-Investigation:

In addition to the information presented in the **Before You Begin** section, what are other *immunization disparities* that Hispanics face? What data can you find to explain these problems? Do these problems extend beyond children into the adult Hispanic community? Why or why not? Lastly, find a bilingual or Spanish immunization schedule you could use as a medical professional.

Section III
Conducting the Eye Exam[1]

Before You Begin

Hispanic children are more at risk to develop blindness or some other type of visual impairment than white children and are less likely to get regular vision checks than black or white children.

Ethnicity also plays a role in vision problems for Hispanic children. Children from this ethnic group are more likely to be diagnosed with astigmatism — blurry vision caused by an irregular curvature of the cornea — than children from any other ethnic group.

Phrases

English	Pronunciation & Spanish
1. Hello I'm (nurse) —-.	*oh-lah soy (ayl ayn-fayr-may-roh / lah ayn-fayr-may-rah) —-.* Hola, soy (el enfermero / la enfermera) —-.[2]
2. Come with me, please.	*bayn kohn-mee-goh pohr fah-bohr.* Ven conmigo, por favor.
3. I am going to test your vision.	*boy ah ah-sayr-tay oon ayk-sah-mayn day lah bee-stah.* Voy a hacerte un examen de la vista.
4. You are going to cover one eye	*bahs ah tah-pahr oon oh-hoh* Vas a tapar un ojo
at a time with this. Like this.	*ah lah bays kohn ay-stoh. ah-see.* a la vez con esto. Así.
5. Stand here and look straight ahead,	*pohn-tay ah-kee ee mee-ray day frayn-tay* Ponte aquí y mira de frente,
please.	*pohr fah-bohr.* por favor.
6. When I tell you, cover your right eye first.	*kwahn-doh tay dee-gah tah-pah ayl oh-hoh day-ray-choh pree-may-roh.* Cuando te diga, tápa el ojo derecho, primero.
7. Now cover your right eye.	*ah-oh-rah tah-pah ayl oh-hoh day-ray-choh.* Ahora, tápa el ojo derecho.
8. You shouldn't be able to see	*noh day-bays poh-dayr bayr* No debes poder ver
anything with your right eye.	*nah-dah kohn ayl oh-hoh day-ray-choh.* nada con el ojo derecho.
9. Don't uncover your right eye	*noh day-stah-pays ayl oh-hoh day-ray-choh* No destapes el ojo derecho
until I tell you to do so.	*ah-stah kay tay loh dee-gah.* hasta que te lo diga.

10. Tell me out loud in which direction	*dee-may ayn bohs **ahl**-tah **ah**-see^ah **dohn**-day* Dime en voz alta hacia dónde
the "feet" of the E are pointing.	*ay-**stahn** lahs pah-**tee**-tahs day lah **lay**-trah ay.* están las patitas de la letra E.[3]
11. Respond with up, down, right or left.	*rray-**spohn**-day kohn ah-**rree**-bah ah-**bah**-hoh day-**ray**-chah oh ees-**kee**^ayr-dah.* Responde con arriba, abajo, derecha o izquierda.[3]
12. Once again, please.	*oh-trah bays pohr fah-**bohr**.* Otra vez, por favor.
13. Now cover your left eye.	*ah-**oh**-rah **tah**-pah ayl **oh**-hoh ees-**kee**^ayr-doh.* Ahora, tápa el ojo izquierdo.
14. You shouldn't be able to see anything	*noh **day**-bays poh-**dayr** bayr **nah**-dah* No debes poder ver nada
with your left eye.	*kohn ayl **oh**-hoh ees-**kee**^ayr-doh.* con el ojo izquierdo.
15. Don't uncover your left eye	*noh day-**stah**-pays ayl **oh**-hoh ees-**kee**^ayr-doh* No destapes el ojo izquierdo
until I tell you to do so.	*ah-stah kay tay loh **dee**-gah.* hasta que te lo diga.
16. We've finished.	*yah **ay**-mohs tayr-mee-**nah**-doh.* Ya hemos terminado.
17. You child (does not have) has	*(soo **nee**-nyoh / **nee**-nyah (noh) **tee**^ay-nay* Su niño / niña (no) tiene
vision problems.	*proh-**blay**-mahs kohn lah **bees**-tah.* problemas con la vista.[4]
18. We need to refer your child	*nay-say-see-**tah**-mohs rray-koh-mayn-**dahr**-lay ah soo **nee**-nyoh / **nee**-nyah ah* Necesitamos recomendarle a su niño / niña
to an eye doctor for a complete	*oon oh-koo-**lee**-stah **pah**-rah ah-**sayr**-lay oon ayk-**sah**-mayn kohm-**play**-toh* a un oculista para hacerle un examen completo
vision test.	*day lah **bee**-stah.* de la vista.[4]

Notes

[1] These instructions are to be used with the *E Eye Exam chart*. Since the *Snellen chart* relies on various letters and the *symbol chart* may have many interpretations in Spanish as well as in English, the *E chart* method requires the exam administrator to recognize very little spoken Spanish vocabulary.

[2] Use *el enfermero* if you are a male nurse and *la enfermera* if you are a female nurse. You may choose to use *el señor, la señora* or *la señorita* with your last name instead. For example: *Soy la señora Smith.*

[3] Repeat necessary phrases.

[4] Use *niño* with a *male child* and *niña* with a *female child*.

Practical Activities III

A) Oral Practice

Instructions: Prepare the following situation and present it to another pair. Remember to switch roles and repeat it again so that each person gets the opportunity to administer the eye exam.

1. Since the eye exam in this chapter is based on the *E Eye Exam Chart*, either find one or create your own for the purposes of practice (for a quick version, draw one or a few on the board far enough apart so that multiple pairs can practice at one time without too many distractions). Then in pairs, take turns administering the eye exam completely in SPANISH. Make sure that the examinee does not do the test perfectly so you get the opportunity to experience a more realistic situation.

B) Matching

Instructions: Match the beginning of each phrase with its proper ending.

1.___ Voy a hacerte . . .		a.	tapa el ojo derecho.
2.___ Ven . . .		b.	terminado.
3.___ Responde con . . .		c.	están las patitas de la letra E.
4.___ No debes poder ver . . .		d.	derecho.
5.___ Cuando te diga . . .		e.	problema con la vista.
6.___ Hemos . . .		f.	mira de frente, por favor.
7.___ Ponte aquí y . . .		g.	un examen de la vista.
8.___ Ahora, tapa el ojo . . .		h.	conmigo, por favor.
9.___ Dime en voz alta hacia dónde . . .		i.	arriba, abajo, derecha o izquierda.
10.___ No tienes ningún . . .		j.	nada con el ojo izquierdo.

Follow-up

Put the completed phrases from exercise **B** in the most logical order possible. Check your order with a class mate to compare. Correct yourself if necessary.

Cyber-Investigation

Searching the internet, find various resources you would be able to give to a Hispanic patient who wanted to read more about vision problems in children. Remember they do not read English and you do not read Spanish. How would you go about gathering this information? How could you make sure it is reliable? Keep a log of these sites for future reference.

Section IV
Conducting the Hearing Exam

Before You Begin

Hispanic children are less likely to have hearing tests due to their limited access to health care. As stated in previous sections, lack of insurance, socioeconomic status, immigration status of parents and/or children, as well as communication barriers often prevent them from either attaining necessary health care and/or understanding the importance and relevance of regular check-ups and health screenings.

Phrases

English	Pronunciation & Spanish
1. Hello I'm (nurse) —.	*oh*-lah soy (ayl ayn-fayr-**may**-roh) —. Hola, soy (el enfermero) —.[1] *oh*-lah soy (lah ayn-fayr-**may**-rah) —. Hola, soy (la enfermera) —.[1]
2. Come with me, please.	*bayn kohn-**mee**-goh pohr fah-**bohr**.* Ven conmigo, por favor.
3. I am going to test your hearing.	*boy ah ah-**sayr**-tay **oo**-nah **proo^ay**-bah day ah^oo-**dee**-see^ohn.* Voy a hacerte una prueba de audición.
4. This is not going to hurt at all.	*noh tay bah ah doh-**layr** pah-rah **nah**-dah.* No te va a doler para nada.
5. Have a seat here, please.	*see^**ayn**-tah-tay ah-**kee** pohr fah-**bohr**.* Siéntate aquí, por favor.
6. Let me tell you what will happen.	*day*-hah-may ayk-splee-**kahr**-tay loh kay bah ah pah-**sahr**. Déjame explicarte lo que va a pasar.
7. You will listen for five different tones.	*bahs ah ays-koo-**chahr** **seen**-koh **toh**-nohs dee-**steen**-tohs.* Vas a escuchar cinco tonos distintos.
8. This is the tool I will use.	*ay*-stay ays ayl ah-pah-**rah**-toh kay boy ah oo-**sahr** Este es el aparato que voy a usar *pah*-rah ah-**sayr**-tay lah **proo^ay**-bah. para hacerte la prueba.
9. I am going to put this in your ear.	*tay loh boy ah poh-**nayr** ayn ayl oh-**ee**-doh.* Te lo voy a poner en el oído.
10. When you hear the tone, raise your index finger.	*kwahn*-doh **oy**-gahs oon **toh**-noh **ahl**-sah Cuando oigas un tono, alza ayl **day**-doh **een**-dee-say. el dedo índice.
11. When you no longer hear the tone,	*kwahn*-doh yah noh **oy**-gas oon **toh**-noh, Cuando ya no oigas un tono,

put your finger down.	*bah*-hah ayl **day**-doh **een**-dee-say. baja el dedo índice.
12. Do not leave your finger raised	noh **day**-hays ayl **day**-doh ahl-**sah**-doh No dejes el dedo alzado
if you no longer hear the tone.	see yah noh **oy**-ays ayl **toh**-noh. si ya no oyes el tono.
13. It's important you follow these	ays eem-pohr-**tahn**-tay say-**gheer ay**-stahs Es importante seguir estas
instructions (strictly) so	een-strook-**see^oh**-nays (ay-streek-tah-**mayn**-tay) **pah**-rah kay instrucciones (estríctamente) para que
the results will be correct.	lohs rray-sool-**tah**-dohs say^ahn koh-**rrayk**-tohs. los resultados sean correctos.
14. I'm sorry, we need to repeat the test.	loh **see^ayn**-toh, nay-say-see-**tah**-mohs rray-pay-**teer** lah **proo^ay**-bah. Lo siento, necesitamos repetir la prueba.
15. Good, we're done.	bee^ayn **ay**-mohs tayr-mee-**nah**-doh. Bien, hemos terminado.
16. You child (does not have) has	soo **nee**-nyoh / **nee**-nyah (noh) **tee^ay**-nay Su niño / niña (no) tiene
a hearing problem.	proh-**blay**-mahs kohn lah ah^oo-dee-**see^ohn**. problemas con la audición.[2]
17. We need to refer your child	nay-say-**see-tah**-mohs rray-koh-mayn-**dahr**-lay ah soo **nee**-nyoh / **nee**-nyah Necesitamos recomendarle a su niño / niña
to an audiologist for	ah oon ah^oo-dee-**oh**-loh-goh **pah**-rah a un audiólogo para
a complete hearing test.	ah-**sayr**-lay oon ayk-**sah**-mayn kohm-**play**-toh day lah ah^oo-dee-**see^ohn**. hacerle un examen completo de la audición.[2]

Notes

[1] Use *el enfermero* if you are a male nurse and *la enfermera* if you are a female nurse. You may choose to use *el señor, la señora* or *la señorita* with your last name instead. For example: *Soy la señora Smith.*

[2] Use *niño* with a *male child* and *niña* with a *female child.*

Practical Activities IV

A) Oral Practice

Introduction: In groups of two or three (possible roles may include *nurse, doctor, parent, child, etc.*), act out the following situations according to the information you are asked to provide. Recreate each situation until each person or group member has had the opportunity to play each role.

1. The nurse must introduce him/herself to the child and have the child (and parent) follow him/her back to the testing room. The nurse tells the child (s)he is going to have a hearing test, then begins to explain what will happen, shows the child the machine and earphones.
2. The nurse instructs the child on what to do and what not do when (s)he hears the various tones. *(Post-test)* The nurse concludes by telling the child the test is over. The nurse then tells the parent there are hearing problems and that the child will need to see a hearing specialist.

B) Sequencing

Instructions: Without referring back to the chapter, number the phrases in this dialogue according to what their proper order should be. Translate the dialogue after you have sequenced them then check your answers with a classmate. Not all phrases from the chapter have been included.

___ - Ven conmigo, por favor. _____

___ - Déjame explicarte lo que va a pasar. _____

___ - Voy a hacerte una prueba de audición. _____

___ - Cuando ya no oigas un tono, baja el dedo índice. _____

___ - Siéntate aquí, por favor. _____

___ - Es importante seguir estas instrucciones para que los resultados sean correctos. _____

_____

___ - Lo siento, necesitamos repetir la prueba. _____

___ - Cuando oigas un tono, alza el dedo índice. _____

___ - Vas a escuchar cinco tonos distintos._____

___ - Hola, soy el enfermo. _____

Cyber-Investigation

Deaf and hearing-impaired English speakers already face many obstacles here in the United States. Imagine, a deaf or severely hearing-impaired monolingual Spanish-speaking child that has recently arrived in the United States. What challenges would he or she face? What challenges would the family face if all members spoke only Spanish as well? Are there resources available for persons in such cases? What are they and how do they help?

Chapter 9

Assessing the Patient's Problem

Section I
Preliminary Questions
and Pain Assessment

Before You Begin

Another cultural difference you may come across is the manner in which Hispanics manage pain. When polled, health care professionals frequently comment that their Hispanic patients appear to experience less pain, even when suffering from severe illnesses and accidents. This can be attributed to the cultural difference in which they react to pain coupled with an inadequate assessment of the pain itself. However, when Hispanic patients were asked to rate their pain on a chart or scale, health care providers observed a noticeable difference between the perceived pain and the true pain felt by the patient.

The use of home remedies *(remedios caseros / rray-may-dee^ohs kah-say-rohs)*, or *folk medicine*, is more common in the Hispanic culture than in U.S. culture and is often used to treat minor illnesses. Therefore, when health care is limited or not easily accessible, a Hispanic may seek out the assistance of a *curandero (koo-rahn-day-roh)* — or folk healer. Although belief in such treatments may be perceived as only belonging to poor, unacculturated Hispanics, the fact is that sometimes educated persons will rely on this practice (known as *el curanderismo / ayl koo-rahn-day-rees-moh)*. However, a patient may not readily confess to having employed such techniques, since they may see it as being culturally unnacceptable to U.S. health care professionals. The assistance provided by the folk healer may not only serve as alternative treatment for medical problems but also for problems associated with psychological disorders. Likewise, it is important to keep in mind that folk healers are likely to have been consulted before medical professionals are consulted for treatment. Finally, some patients may also believe their condition to be supernatural in origin.

In Hispanic countries, pharmacists *(farmacólogos / fahr-mah-koh-loh-gohs)* are often the first medical professionals consulted about a health-related problem. The training a Hispanic pharmacist recieves is often in-depth, thus allowing him/her to administer shots and prescribe medicines without a physician's written prescription. In some Latin American countries, there are even stores similar to these pharmacies *(farmacias / fahr-mah-see^ahs)* called *botánicas (boh-tah-nee-kahs)* where herbal remedies are sold to be used as cures for various ailments.

Phrases

English	Pronunciation & Spanish
1. I'm Dr. —.	*soy ayl dohk-tohr* —. Soy el doctor —.[1] *soy lah dohk-toh-rah.* Soy la doctora —.[1]

2. I'm nurse —.	*soy ayl ayn-fayr-**may**-roh / soy lah ayn-fayr-**may**-rah—.* Soy el enfermero / la enfermera—.[1]
3. Are you feeling bad today?	*say **see^ayn**-tay mahl oy?* ¿Se siente mal hoy?
4. How many days have you felt bad?	***kwahn**-tohs **dee**-ahs **ah**-say kay say **see^ayn**-tay mahl?* ¿Cuántos días hace que se siente mal?[2]
5. Show me with your finger where	*say-**nyah**-lay kohn ayl **day**-doh **dohn**-day* Señale con el dedo dónde
the problem is.	*ay-**stah** ayl proh-**blay**-mah.* está el problema.[5]
6. Do you feel pain (now)?	***see^ayn**-tay doh-**lohr** (ah-**oh**-rah)?* ¿Siente dolor (ahora)?
7. Have you had any pain?	*ah sayn-**tee**-doh doh-**lohr**?* ¿Ha sentido dolor?
8. Do you feel worse in . . .	*say **see^ayn**-tay pay-**ohr** pohr . . .* ¿Se siente peor por . . .
the morning?	*lah mah-**nyah**-nah?* la mañana?
the afternoon?	*lah **tahr**-day?* la tarde?
the evening/at night?	*lah **noh**-chay?* la noche?
9. Show me with your finger	*say-**nyah**-lay kohn ayl **day**-doh* Señale con el dedo
where you feel the pain.	***dohn**-day **see^ayn**-tay ayl doh-**lohr**.* dónde siente el dolor.[5]
10. Is the pain . . .	*ays ayl doh-**lohr** . . .* ¿Es el dolor . . .
strong/severe?	***fwayr**-tay?* fuerte?
sharp?	*ah-**goo**-doh?* agudo?
mild?	***lay**-bay?* leve?
dull?	***sohr**-doh?* sordo?
persistent?	*payr-see-**stayn**-tay?* persistente?
burning?	*ahr-**dee^ayn**-tay?* ardiente?

throbbing?	*pahl-pee-**tahn**-tay?* palpitante?
localized?	*loh-kahl-lee-**sah**-doh?* localizado?

11. Will you show me on this scale	*may say-**nyah**-lay ayn **ay**-stah ay-**skah**-lah* ¿Me señala en esta escala
of one to ten the severity of the pain?	*day **oo**-noh ah dee^ays lah say-bay-ree-**dahd** dayl doh-**lohr**?* de uno a diez la severidad del dolor?[3]
12. Does the pain radiate?	*say **koh**-rray ayl doh-**lohr**?* ¿Se corre el dolor?
13. Show me from where to where.	***mway**-stray-may day **dohn**-day ah **dohn**-day.* Muéstreme de dónde a dónde.[5]
14. Are you taking any medication?	*ay-**stah** toh-**mahn**-doh may-dee-**see**-nah?* ¿Está tomando medicina?
15. Have you taken any medicine?	*ah toh-**mah**-doh may-dee-**see**-nah?* ¿Ha tomado medicina?
16. Will you write the name here?	*may ay-**skree**-bay ayl **nohm**-bray ah-**kee**?* ¿Me escribe el nombre aquí?[2]
17. Are you taking any home remedies?	*ay-**stah** toh-**mahn**-doh ahl-**goon** rray-**may**-dee^oh kah-**say**-roh?* ¿Está tomando algún remedio casero?
18. Have you taken any home remedies?	*ha toh-**mah**-doh ahl-**goon** rray-**may**-dee^oh kah-**say**-roh?* ¿Ha tomado algún remedio casero?[4]
19. What is it?	*kwahl ays?* ¿Cuál es?[2]

Notes

[1] Use *el doctor* or *el enfermero* if you are a male and *la doctora* or *la enfermera* if you are a female.

[2] Have patients write this answer on a piece of paper for you.

[3] See the *Pain Scale/Escala de dolor* found in the **APPENDIX** for this section.

[4] A list of common *FOLK REMEDIES* have been included in the **APPENDIX** for this section.

[5] You may elect to use the *BODY DIAGRAM* provided in the **APPENDIX** for this chapter. Remember, you need not be able to say the names of the body parts in Spanish in order to use the chart. However, they can be found in Chapter 18.

Practical Activities I

A) Oral Practice

Instructions: In pairs, using the pain scale referenced in the **NOTES** section of this chapter, conduct a *preliminary pain assessment* according to the guidelines provided for each situation. Before beginning, the patient should note his/her anticipated responses. During the course of the assessment, the person carrying out the assessment should be sure to note the patient's reponses. When you are done, verify your notes with your partner's anticipated responses for accurracy. Switch roles with your partner and recreate each situation. Remember to communicate in SPANISH ONLY! You may elect to use the *BODY DIAGRAM* found in the Appendix for this chapter as a visual aid.

1. The doctor/nurse introduces him/herself and asks if the patient feels bad and for how long (s)he has felt this way. The doctor/nurse asks the patient to point out the problem and asks if there is currently any pain. The doctor/nurse asks when the pain is worse and then offers the patient options to describe the pain. Finally the doctor/nurse asks the patient to show him/her on the *pain scale* the severity of the pain.
2. The doctor/nurse asks the patient if (s)he is in pain, how bad it is and where it begins and ends. The doctor/nurse then asks if the patient has been treating the pain, how and with what. Doctor/Nurse thens asks the patient to write the names of any supplements and home remedies (s)he has taken (*see the list of common FOLK REMEDIES in the appendix for this section*).

B) ¡Qué dolor! (What pain!) — Part 1

Instructions: Various patients you are seeing today are in pain and are describing it to you, the medical professional. As you listen (actually, read it below in Spanish) to what they are saying, you write notes in each patient's chart in English.

Patient	Chart
Sr. Rodriguez: "El dolor es peor por la mañana. Es agudo y muy fuerte . . . Sí, 3 aspirinas".	Notes:
Sra. Santos: "El dolor es persistente y palpitante. No es ardiente . . . No he tomado medicina".	Notes:
Srta. Bautista: "Sí, he tomado algún remedio casero - el te de canela . . . El dolor es peor por la noche y es sordo y localizado".	Notes:

Cyber-Investigation

It is not uncommon for Hispanics to turn to folk medicine for treatment of illnesses and afflictions before consulting a health care provider. Also, this tends to be more prevelant among illegal Hispanics. Why is folk medicine still popular in the Hispanic population? Why would illegal Hispanics be more likely to seek out this alternative treatment? Give 2 to 3 popular examples of Hispanic folk remedies not mentioned in the Appendix.

Section II
General Diagnostic Questions

Before You Begin

Hispanics with little or no education at all may explain their discomforts from a cutural perspective or in more general terms. The term *ataque (ah-**tah**-kay)* is used to describe what many people would reference as an *episode*. Also, these descriptions may be based on superstitious beliefs, such as the *mal de ojo (mahl day **oh**-hoh)* or the evil eye. Whatever the case may be, remember not to pass judgement on their belief system as these are very real descriptions of the condition to that person.

Remember that the Hispanic culture places great emphasis on respect. Therefore, one of the best methods to build patient trust and establish rapport is to request the Hispanic patient's permission before beginning an exam or asking personal health-related questions. The phrase *"Con su permiso" (kohn soo payr-**mee**-soh)*, meaning *"With your permission,"* would be highly appropriate for such situations.

Phrases

English	Pronunciation & Spanish
1. Have you lost weight recently?	*ah bah-**hah**-doh day **pay**-soh rray-see^ayn-tay-**mayn**-tay?* ¿Ha bajado de peso recientemente?
2. Have you gained weight recently?	*ah ah^oo-mayn-**tah**-doh day **pay**-soh rray-see^ayn-tay-**mayn**-tay?* ¿Ha aumentado de peso recientemente?
3. Respond "now," "before," or "no"	*rray-**spohn**-dah ah-**oh**-rah **ahn**-tays oh noh* Responda "ahora," "antes," o "no"
to the following questions, please.	*ah lahs pray-**goon**-tahs see-**ghee**^ayn-tays pohr fah-**bohr**.* a las preguntas siguientes, por favor.[1]
4. Do you or have you had any . . .	*tee^**ay**-nay oh ah tay-**nee**-doh . . .* ¿Tiene o ha tenido . . .
nausea?	*nah^**oo**-see-ahs?* nauseas?
dizziness?	*mah-**ray**-ohs?* mareos?
fainting spells?	*days-**mah**-yohs?* desmayos?
chills?	*ay-skah-loh-**free**-ohs?* escalofríos?
fever?	*fee^**ay**-bray?* fiebre?
rash?	*sahl-poo-**yee**-doh?* salpullido?
chest pain?	*doh-**lohr** ayn ayl **pay**-choh?* dolor en el pecho?

headache?	*doh-**lohr** day kah-**bay**-sah?* dolor de cabeza?
numbness?	*ayn-too-may-see-**mee**^**ayn**-toh?* entumecimiento?[2]
5. Do you or have you had problems . . .	***tee**^**ay**-nay oh ah tay-**nee**-doh proh-**blay**-mahs ahl . . .* ¿Tiene o ha tenido problemas al . . .
sleeping?	*door-**meer**?* dormir?
breathing?	*rray-spee-**rahr**?* respirar?
6. Do you feel . . .	*say **see**^**ayn**-tay . . .* ¿Se siente . . .
tired?	*kahn-**sah**-doh/dah?* cansado/a?[3]
weak?	***day**-beel?* débil?

Notes:

[1] Use this statement throughout the *diagnostic questions sections* in order to easily understand patient responses.

[2] Another term for *entumecimiento* is *adormecimiento (ah-dohr-may-see-**mee**^ayn-toh)*.

[3] Remember to use *cansado* when talking to a *male patient* and *cansada* when talking to a *female patient*.

Practical Activities II

A) Oral Practice

Instructions: Individually, prepare responses to all of the General Diagnostic Questions. Then, in pairs, have one person play the role of health care provider and the other person, the patient. The health care provider will then introduce him/herself and let the patient know that (s)he will be asked some questions (remember to use the courtesy expression *Con su permiso*). Continue by asking the patient the General Diagnostic Questions and charting all responses. After all questions have been asked, check the actual answers against the charted responses for accuracy. Then switch roles and repeat the process. Vary your responses so that you become acquainted with the possible responses provided.

B) ¡Qué dolor! (What pain!) — Part 2

Instructions: You are now asking the same three patients questions about their general physical state. As you listen (actually, read it below in Spanish) to what they are saying, you write notes in each patient's chart in English.

Health Care Provider/Patient Dialogue	Chart
HP: ¿Ha bajado de peso recientemente?	Notes:
Sr. Rodriguez: Sí.	
HP: ¿Tiene o ha tenido fiebre y salpullido?	
Sr. Rodriguez: Fiebre, antes, salpullido, no.	
HP: ¿Tiene dolor en el pecho?	
Sr. Rodriguez: Sí, tengo mucho dolor en el pecho.	
HP: ¿Tiene problemas al respirar?	
Sr. Rodriguez: Ahora, sí.	
HP: ¿Ha aumentado de peso recientemente?	Notes:
Sra. Santos: Un poco.	
HP: ¿Tiene o ha tenido desmayos y dolor de cabeza?	
Sra. Santos: Sí, desmayos y dolor antes y ahora.	
HP: ¿Se siente cansada?	
Sra. Santos: Cansada, no. Débil, sí.	
HP: ¿Tiene o ha tenido adormeciento?	Notes:
Srta. Bautista: Sí, ahora . . . en las piernas (my legs).	
HP: ¿Tiene o ha tenido problemas al respirar?	
Srta. Bautista: No.	
HP: ¿Se siente débil o cansada?	
Srta. Bautista: No.	

Cyber-Investigation

The concept of *mal de ojo (mahl day oh-hoh)* is very prevelant among young and old Hispanics alike. What information can you find as to why superstition is such an integral part of Hispanic culture? How did this come about and why does it continue even today? Search the Internet for information and facts. Site three additional examples of such supersitious beliefs of the Hispanic community.

Section III
Sensory Organs : Mouth, Throat, Nose, Ears, Eyes and Skin

Before You Begin

In some rural areas of Hispanic countries, the words *cáncer* (**kahn**-sayr) and *lepra* (**lay**-prah) may be used out of their literal context to describe certain serious skin problems. For example, *cáncer* may refer to any severe infection of the skin, including gangrene and infected wounds. The word *lepra* may reference any sort of sore, such as boils or ringworm, as well as allergic skin reactions that spread.

Phrases

English	Pronunciation & Spanish
1. Do your gums or mouth bleed?	*lay **sahn**-grahn lahs ayn-**see**-ahs?* ¿Le sagran las encías?
2. Does your mouth bleed?	*lay **sahn**-grah lah **boh**-kah?* ¿Le sangra la boca?
3. Does . . . feel sore/hurt?	***lay dway**-lay . . .* ¿Le duele . . .
your tongue	*lah **layn**-gwah?* la lengua?
any other part of your mouth	***oh**-trah **pahr**-tay day lah **boh**-kah?* otra parte de la boca?
4. Does your tongue feel . . .	***tee^ay**-nay lah **layn**-gwah . . .* ¿Tiene la lengua . . .
swollen?	*een-**chah**-dah?* hinchada?
thick?	***groo^ay**-sah?* gruesa?
rough?	***ah**-spay-rah?* áspera?
5. Does your throat . . .	*lay . . . lah gahr-**gahn**-tah?* ¿Le . . . la garganta?
hurt?	***dway**-lay* duele
feel scratchy?	***pee**-kah* pica
6. Do you have problems swallowing?	***tee^ay**-nay proh-**blay**-mahs ahl trah-**gahr**?* ¿Tiene problemas al tragar?
7. Are you or have you been hoarse?	***tee^ay**-nay oh ah tay-**nee**-doh lah bohs **rrohn**-kah?* ¿Tiene o ha tenido la voz ronca?

8. Have you noticed any lumps in your neck?

*ah noh-**tah**-doh ahl-**goo**-nahs boh-**lee**-tahs ayn ayl **kway**-yoh?*
¿Ha notado algunas bolitas en el cuello?

9. Have you noticed any swelling in the

*ah noh-**tah**-doh ahl-**goo**-nah een-chah-**sohn** day lahs*
¿Ha notado alguna hinchazón de las

glands of your neck?

*glahn-doo-lahs ayn ayl **kway**-yoh?*
glándulas en el cuello?

10. Does your nose feel clogged?

*tee^ay-nay lah nah-**rees** tah-**pah**-dah?*
¿Tiene la nariz tapada?

11. Does your nose bleed?

*lay **sahn**-grah lah nah-**rees**?*
¿Le sangra la nariz?

12. Can you breath through your nose?

*pway-day rray-spee-**rahr** pohr lah nah-**rees**?*
¿Puede respirar por la nariz?

13. Do you have problems hearing?

*tee^ay-nay proh-**blay**-mahs ahl oh-**eer**?*
¿Tiene problemas al oír?

14. Do you get ear infections?

*soo-fray day een-fayk-**see^oh**-nays dayl oh-**ee**-doh?*
¿Sufre de infecciones del oído?

15. Do you have a ringing in your ears?

*lay **soom**-bahn lohs oh-**ee**-dohs?*
¿Le zumban los oídos?

16. Will you show me which one?

*may say-**nyah**-lah kwahl ays?*
¿Me señala cuál es?

17. Do your ears run?

*lay **sah**-lay **ahl**-goh day lohs oh-**ee**-dohs?*
¿Le sale algo de los oídos?

18. Do you have vision problems?

*tee^ay-nay proh-**blay**-mahs kohn lah **bee**-stah?*
¿Tiene problemas con la vista?

19. Do you wear . . .

oo-sah . . .
¿Usa . . .

glasses?

*ahn-tay-**oh**-hohs?*
anteojos?[2]

contact lenses?

*layn-tays day kohn-**tahk**-toh?*
lentes de contacto?

20. Always or sometimes?

*see^aym-pray oh ah **bay**-says?*
¿Siempre o a veces?

21. For . . .

pah-rah . . .
¿Para . . .

seeing close up?

*bayr day **sayr**-kah?*
ver de cerca?

seeing far away?

*bayr day **lay**-hohs?*
ver de lejos?

reading?

*lay-**ayr**?*
leer?

22. Do both eyes . . .	*lay . . . lohs dohs oh-hohs?* ¿Le . . . los dos ojos?
hurt?	*dway-layn* duelen
burn?	*ahr-dayn* arden
itch?	*pee-kahn* pican
23. Do you have . . . vision?	*tee^ay-nay lah bee-stah . . .* ¿Tiene la vista . . .
double	*doh-blay?* doble?
blurred	*boh-rroh-sah?* borrosa?
cloudy	*noo-blah-dah?* nublada?
24. Did anything get in your eye?	*lay ayn-troh ahl-goh ayn ayl oh-hoh?* ¿Le entró algo en el ojo?
25. Do you have a rash?	*tee^ay-nay ahl-goon sahl-poo-yee-doh?* ¿Tiene algún salpullido?
26. Will you show me, please?	*may loh mways-trah pohr fah-bohr?* ¿Me lo muestra, por favor?
27. Were you bitten by an insect?	*lay ah pee-kah-doh oon een-sayk-toh?* ¿Le ha picado un insecto?
28. Have you eaten anything different lately?	*ah koh-mee-doh ahl-go dee-fay-rayn-tay rray-see^ayn-tay-mayn-tay?* ¿Ha comido algo diferente recientemente?
29. Have you used a . . .	*ah oo-sah-doh oon . . .* ¿Ha usado un . . .
new type of soap?	*hah-bohn noo^ay-boh?* jabón nuevo?
new brand of detergent?	*day-tayr-hayn-tay noo^ay-boh?* detergente nuevo?
30. Do you suffer from chronic skin diseases?	*soo-fray day ayn-fayr-may-dah-days kroh-nee-kahs day lah pee^ayl?* ¿Sufre de enfermedades crónicas de la piel?
31. Psoriasis?	*soh-ree^ah-sees?* ¿Psoriasis?[1]
32. Seborrhoea?	*say-boh-rray-ah?* ¿Seborrea?

Notes

[1] The popular lay term for *Psoriasis* is *Sarna (**sahr**-nah)*. This is also the word for *scabies*. However, this term may be offensive since many times it erroneously associates the disease with unkempt, lower-class people. Use it only if the term provided is not understood.

[2] Other popular words for *glasses* are *lentes (**layn**-tays)*, *gafas (**gah**-fahs)* and *espejuelos (ay-spay-**whay**-lohs)*.

Practical Activities III

A) Oral Practice — Reverse Conversation

Instructions: Individually, write 1 through 32 on a sheet of paper. Then, go through all 32 questions from this chapter and write down a simple, logical response for each one in SPANISH (do not write out the question). Write your name in the top right-hand corner of the paper and trade with a partner. Have that person write his/her name under yours.

Form pairs and have one person play the role of health care provider and the other person, the patient. The health care provider will ask the patient the questions from this chapter in order while the patient supplies the pre-written response. However, this time, instead of the health care provider making notes about the patient's responses, the patient will be making notes about the question (s)he has been asked.

For example:

Health care Provider asks the first question - 1. ¿Le sangran las encías?
Patient reads prepared response aloud from answer sheet - 1. Sí.
Patient notates question in English - 1. Sí - Do your gums bleed?

Health care Provider asks the second question - 2. ¿Le sangra la boca?
Patient reads prepared response aloud from answer sheet - 1. No.
Patient notates question in English - 1. No - Does your mouth bleed?
etc.

If short on time, switch roles half-way through. After both persons have had the chance to play both roles, give the answer sheet back to its originator. This person will then check to see if the notes made by the patient regarding the question being asked were correct.

B) ¡Qué dolor! (What pain!) — Part 3

Instructions: You are continuing the diagnostic questioning of the same three patients from the previous chapter, but this time regarding their Sensory Organs. As you listen (actually, read it below in Spanish) to what they are saying, you write notes in each patient's chart in English.

Another option is have two people read the conversations aloud while the rest of the class listens and makes notes without the use of the text. Afterwards, everyone will compare their notes with another person before consulting the text for accuracy.

Health Care Provider/Patient Dialogue	Chart
HP: ¿Le duele la lengua?	Notes:
Sr. Rodriguez: No. La garganta, sí.	
HP: ¿Ha notado algunas bolitas en el cuello?	
Sr. Rodriguez: Sí.	
HP: ¿Tiene problemas al oír?	
Sr. Rodriguez: Un poco.	
HP: ¿Le sale algo de los oídos?	
Sr. Rodriguez: Sí, por la noche.	

Exercise continues on next page

Health Care Provider/Patient Dialogue	**Chart**
HP: ¿Tiene la lengua hinchada?	Notes:
Sra. Santos: Sí.	
HP: ¿Tiene la nariz tapada?	
Sra. Santos: Sí.	
HP: ¿Le sangra la nariz?	
Sra. Santos: No.	
HP: ¿Le ha picado un insecto?	
Sra. Santos: Sí.	
HP: ¿Le entró algo en el ojo?	Notes:
Srta. Bautista: Sí, el derecho (the right one).	
HP: ¿Tiene la vista doble, borrosa o nublada?	
Srta. Bautista: Doble y nublada.	
HP: ¿Le arden los dos ojos?	
Srta. Bautista: No. Pican mucho.	

Section IV
Cardiopulmonary System

Before You Begin

The popularity of tobacco use among Hispanics places them at high risk for cardiovascular disease. A national study showed Hispanic males smoking more than Hispanic females, though the Hispanic females smoked less than females from other ethnic groups. Unfortunately, the same study also revealed a trend in the increase of smoking among Hispanic teenagers over the past 30 years.

Lung cancer is the leading cause of cancer-related deaths among Hispanics.

Phrases

English	Pronunciation & Spanish
1. Have you ever had an electrocardiogram?	*lay ahn **ay**-choh oon ay-layk-troh-kahr-dee^oh-**grah**-mah ahl-**goo**-nah bays?* ¿Le han hecho un electrocardiograma alguna vez?
2. Do you get palpitations	***tee^ay**-nay pahl-pee-tah-**see^oh**-nays* ¿Tiene palpitaciones
(accompanied by pain)?	*(kohn doh-**lohr**)?* (con dolor)?
3. Do you have or have you had	***tee^ay**-nay oh ah tay-**nee**-doh* ¿Tiene o ha tenido
irregular heartbeats?	*lah-**tee**-dohs ee-rray-goo-**lah**-rays?* latidos irregulares?
4. Do you have a heart murmur?	***tee^ay**-nay oon moor-**moo**-yoh ayn ayl koh-rah-**sohn**?* ¿Tiene un murmullo en el corazón?
5. Have you ever had a heart attack?	*ah tay-**nee**-doh oon ah-**tah**-kay kahr-**dee**-ah-koh ahl-**goo**-nah bays?* ¿Ha tenido un ataque cardíaco alguna vez?
6. Do you have or have you had	***tee^ay**-nay oh ah tay-**nee**-doh* ¿Tiene o ha tenido
chest pains?	*doh-**loh**-rays ayn ayl **pay**-choh?* dolores en el pecho?
7. Are you in pain now?	***noh**-tah ahl-**goon** doh-**lohr** ah-**oh**-rah?* ¿Nota algún dolor ahora?
8. Point with your finger where	*say-**nyah**-lay-may kohn ayl **day**-doh **dohn**-day* Señáleme con el dedo dónde
you normally feel the pain.	*see^ayn-tay ayl doh-**lohr** nohr-mahl-**mayn**-tay.* siente el dolor normalmente.
9. Does the pain last long?	*lay **doo**-rah ayl doh-**lohr** moo-choh **tee^aym**-poh?* ¿Le dura el dolor mucho tiempo?

10. How often do you have pain?

*kohn kay fray-**kwayn**-see^ah **tee^ay**-nay doh-**lohr**?*
¿Con qué frecuencia tiene dolor?[1]

11. Does the pain start gradually

*aym-**pee^ay**-sah ayl doh-**lohr** poh-koh ah **poh**-koh*
¿Empieza el dolor poco a poco

or suddenly?

*oh day rray-**payn**-tay?*
o de reprente?

12. Show me with your finger

*say-**nyah**-lay-me kohn ayl **day**-doh **ah**-stah*
Señáleme con el dedo hasta

where the pain radiates.

***dohn**-day say lay **koh**-rray ayl doh-**lohr**.*
dónde se le corre el dolor.

13. Do you exercise regularly?

***ah**-say ay-hayr-**see**-see^oh rray-goo-lahr-**mayn**-tay?*
¿Hace ejercicio regularmente?

14. Do you have difficulties breathing?

***tee^ay**-nay dee-fee-kool-**tahd** ahl rray-spee-**rahr**?*
¿Tiene dificultad al respirar?

15. Do you wheeze?

***tee^ay**-nay lah rray-spee-rah-**see^ohn** hah-day-**ahn**-tay?*
¿Tiene la respiración jadeante?

16. Do you have or have you had

***tee^ay**-nay oh ah tay-**nee**-doh*
¿Tiene o ha tenido

frequent colds?

*rrays-**free^ah**-dohs fray-**kwayn**-tays?*
resfriados frecuentes?

17. Do you cough a lot?

***toh**-say **moo**-choh?*
¿Tose mucho?

18. Does it hurt to cough?

*lay **dway**-lay ahl toh-**sayr**?*
¿Le duele al toser?

19. Is there a position that makes

*ah^ee ahl-**goo**-nah poh-see-**see^ohn** kay*
¿Hay alguna posición que

your breathing . . .

*lay . . . lah rray-spee-rah-**see^ohn**?*
le . . . la respiración?

easier?

*fah-see-**lee**-tay*
facilite

harder?

*dee-fee-**kool**-tay*
dificulte

20. Do you bring up (a lot of) phlegm?

*lay **sah**-lay (**moo**-chah) **flay**-mah?*
¿Le sale (mucha) flema?

21. Is it . . .

ays . . .
¿Es . . .

black?

***nay**-grah?*
negra?

brown?

*mah-**rrohn**?*
marrón?

(dark) red?	*rroh-jah (oh-skoo-rah)?* roja (oscura)?
yellow?	*ah-mah-ree-yah?* amarilla?
green?	*bayr-day?* verde?
gray?	*grees?* gris?
white?	*blahn-kah?* blanca?
clear?	*klah-rah?* clara?
22. Have you ever had asthma, TB, and/or emphysema?	*ah soo-free-doh day ahs-mah,* ¿Ha sufrido de asma, *too-bayr-koo-loh-sees ee / oh ayn-fee-say-mah?* tuberculosis, y / o enfisema?
23. Do you or have you smoked?	*foo-mah oh ah foo-mah-doh?* ¿Fuma o ha fumado?
24. Have you completely stopped smoking?	*ah day-hah-doh day foo-mahr pohr kohm-play-toh?* ¿Ha dejado de fumar por completo?

Notes

[1] Use the *FREQUENCY CHART* found in the **APPENDIX** for this chapter. For questions to assess the severity of pain see **APPENDIX: Chapter 9 - Assessing the Patient's Problem - Preliminary Questions/Pain Assessment** and use it in conjunction with the *PAIN SCALE* found in the **APPENDIX** for that chapter.

Practical Activities IV

A) Oral Practice

Instructions: Invidually, divide a sheet of paper into three columns. Label the first column *My Responses* and number it 1-24. Then, label the second column *Patient 1 Responses* and number it 1-24 as well. Lastly, label the last column *Patient 2 Responses* and number it 1-24. Go through all 24 questions from this chapter and write down a simple, logical response for each one in SPANISH only under the first column labeled *My Responses* (do not write out the question), leaving the other columns blank.

Form a group of three, in which each person is designated either as **A**, **B** or **C**. Start with **A** being the patient, and **B** and **C** being the health care providers. **B** will use the book and read each question aloud to the patient. **C** only has his/her paper but no book and should not be able to see the phrases that **B** is reading. The patient, **A**, will respond according to his/her prewritten answers under the column titled *My Responses*. As **A** answers, **B** and **C** note **A**'s responses in ENGLISH under the column titled *Patient 1 Responses* beside of the corresponding question number. Not only should the response be noted but written in the form of a short, concise note.

For example:

> *B asks:* ¿Le han hecho un electrocardiograma alguna vez?
> *A responds:* Sí
> *B and C write:* Patient has had an EKG.

To minimize confusion, **B** may say the number of the question being asked so **C** does not loose track. After the questions have all been asked, **C** should read aloud his/her responses as **B** and **A** check them for accuracy. Change roles so that **A** is **B**, **B** is **C** and **C** is **A**. Repeat the process again. If time permits, go through the role play a third time, again changing roles so that each group member has been a health care provider twice and a patient once.

If short on time, have the health care providers share the asking of the questions with one person asking 1-12 and the second person asking 13-24. When using this option, remember, whomever is not asking the question may not use the text.

B) ¡Qué dolor! (What pain!) - Part 4

Instructions: You are asking your patients diagnostic questions about their Cardiopulmonary System. As you listen (actually, read it below in Spanish) to what they are saying, you write notes in each patient's chart in English.

Another option is to have two people read the conversations aloud while the rest of the class listens and makes notes without the use of the text. Afterwards, everyone will compare their notes with another person before consulting the text for accuracy.

Health Care Provider/Patient Dialogue	Chart
HP: ¿Tiene palpitaciones con dolor?	Notes:
Sr. Rodriguez: Sí pero sin (without) dolor.	
HP: ¿Tiene o ha tenido latidos irregulares?	
Sr. Rodriguez: Sí.	
HP: ¿Con qué frecuencia?	
Sr. Rodriguez: Dos veces a la semana. *(see FREQUENCY CHART)*	
HP: ¿Tose mucho?	
Sr. Rodriguez: No.	

Exercise continues on next page

Health Care Provider/Patient Dialogue	Chart
HP: ¿Tiene dificultad al respirar? Sra. Santos: Sí. *HP: ¿Tiene la respiración jadeante?* Sra. Santos: Ahora, no. Antes, sí. *HP: ¿Hace ejercicio regularmente?* Sra. Santos: Tres veces a la semana. *(see FRE-QUENCY CHART)*	Notes:
HP: ¿Ha sufrido de asma, tuberculosis y/o en-fisema? Srta. Bautista: Asma. *HP: ¿Le sale flema?* Srta. Bautista: Sí. Mucho. *HP: ¿Es amarilla o verde?* Srta. Bautista: No. Clara.	Notes:

Section V
Gastrointestinal System

Before You Begin

Eating habits of Hispanics are different than those of the typical U.S. American. Not only does the type of food vary greatly from country to country and region to region but meal times are often different as well. For many Hispanics, *lunch (el almuerzo / ayl ahl-moo^ayr-soh)* is the primary meal of the day while *breakfast (el desayuno / ayl day-sah^ee-oo-noh)* and *dinner (la cena / lah say-nah)* are much lighter. Many times, dinner is also eaten quit late in the evening. As a direct result of their diet, gastrointestinal problems and a high risk for the development of gallstones are commonplace among Hispanics.

Phrases

English	Pronunciation & Spanish
1. Are there foods that disagree with you?	*ah^ee koh-**mee**-dahs kay lay **kah^ee**-gahn mahl?* ¿Hay comidas que le caigan mal?
2. Do you eat greasy or fried foods?	***toh**-mah koh-**mee**-dahs grah-**soh**-sahs oh **free**-tahs?* ¿Toma comidas grasosas o fritas?
3. Do you suffer from . . .	***soo**-fray day . . .* ¿Sufre de . . .
gas?	*gahs?* gas?
indigestion?	*een-dee-hay-**stee^ohn**?* indigestión?
heartburn?	*ahr-**dohr** day ay-**stoh**-mah-goh?* ardor de estómago?
stomach aches?	*doh-**lohr** day ay-**stoh**-mah-goh?* dolor de estómago?
constipation?	*ayk-stray-nyee-**mee^ayn**-toh?* extreñimiento?
diarrhea?	*dee^ah-**rray**-ah?* diarrea?
cramps?	*kah-**lahm**-brays?* calambres?
4. How often?	*kohn kay fray-**kwayn**-see^ah?* ¿Con qué frecuencia?[1]
5. Normally, . . .	*nohr-mahl-**mayn**-tay* Normalmente, ¿ . . .
before eating?	***ahn**-tays day koh-**mayr**?* antes de comer?

while you're eating?	*mee^ayn-trahs koh-may?* mientras come?
after eating?	*day-spways day koh-mayr?* después de comer?

---

6. Do you drink . . .	*toh-mah . . .* ¿Toma . . .
water?	*ah-gwah?* agua?
soft drinks?	*rray-fray-skohs?* refrescos?
coffee?	*kah-fay rray-goo-lahr?* café regular?
decaffeinated coffee?	*kah-fay days-kah-fay^ee-nah-doh?* café descafeinado?
whole milk?	*lay-chay ayn-tay-rah?* leche entera?
lowfat milk?	*lay-chay bah-hah ayn grah-sah?* leche baja en grasa?
skim milk?	*lay-chay days-nah-tah-dah?* leche desnatada?
beer?	*sayr-bay-sah?* cerveza?
white wine?	*bee-noh blahn-koh?* vino blanco?
red wine?	*bee-noh teen-toh?* vino tinto?
other alcoholic beverages?	*oh-trahs bay-bee-dahs ahl-koh-oh-lee-kahs?* otras bebidas alcohólicas?

---

7. How often do you drink . . .	*kohn kay fray-kwayn-see^ah toh-mah . . .* ¿Con qué frecuencia toma . . . [1]
water?	*ah-gwah?* agua?
soft drinks?	*rray-fray-skohs?* refrescos?
coffee?	*kah-fay rray-goo-lahr?* café regular?
decaffeinated coffee?	*kah-fay days-kah-fay^ee-nah-doh?* café descafeinado?
whole milk?	*lay-chay ayn-tay-rah?* leche entera?

lowfat milk?	*lay*-chay **bah**-hah ayn **grah**-sah? leche baja en grasa?
skim milk?	*lay*-chay days-nah-**tah**-dah? leche desnatada?
beer?	sayr-**bay**-sah? cerveza?
white wine?	**bee**-noh **blahn**-koh? vino blanco?
red wine?	**bee**-noh **teen**-toh? vino tinto?
other alcoholic beverages?	**oh**-trahs bay-**bee**-dahs ahl-koh-**oh**-lee-kahs? otras bebidas alcohólicas?
8. Do you belch a lot?	ay-**rook**-tah **moo**-choh? ¿Eructa mucho?
9. Do you eat breakfast regularly?	**toh**-mah ayl day-sah^ee-**oo**-noh rray-goo-lahr-**mayn**-tay? ¿Toma el desayuno regularmente?
10. Do you eat . . .	**koh**-may . . . ¿Come . . .
red meat?	**kahr**-nay **rroh**-hah? carne roja?
white meat?	**kahr**-nay **blahn**-kah? carne blanca?
fish?	pay-**skah**-doh? pescado?
seafood?	mah-**ree**-skohs? mariscos?
vegetables?	bay-hay-**tah**-lays? vegetales?
fruits?	**froo**-tahs? frutas?
bread and cereals?	pahn ee say-ray-**ah**-lays? pan y cereales?
11. Do you eat late at night?	**koh**-may mwee **tahr**-day pohr lah **noh**-chay? ¿Come muy tarde por la noche?
12. Do you have a bowel movement every day?	bah day **bee**^ayn-tray **toh**-dohs lohs **dee**-ahs? ¿Va de vientre todos los días?[2]
13. Does it hurt when you defecate?	lay **dway**-lay eer day **vee**^ayn-tray (eer dayl dohs)? ¿Le duele ir de vientre (ir del dos)?

14. Have you seen any blood or

mucus in your stool?

ah noh-__tah__-doh __sahn__-gray oh
¿Ha notado sangre o

moo-koh-see-__dahd__ ayn ayl ayk-skray-__mayn__-toh?
mucosidad en el excremento?

Notes

[1] Use the *FREQUENCY CHART* found in the **APPENDIX: Chapter 9 - Assessing the Patient's Problem - Cardiopulmonary System.**

[2] There are numerous ways of stating this phrase, ranging from highly formal to vulgar. This particular one was researched and found to be universally understood without leaning towards harsher terminology. Should this phrase still present a misunderstanding, the phrase *¿Va del dos todos los días? / vah dayl dohs __toh__-dohs lohs __dee__-ahs?* is also commonly used, but takes on a lower linguistic register, though it still avoids any potential vulgarity.

Practical Activities V

A) Oral Practice

Instructions: In pairs, one person will play the role of the health care provider and the other will play the role of the patient. The objective of the health care provider is to obtain the information requested using SPANISH only. Of course, the patient will respond only in SPANISH as well. Remember, all of these patients are new and do not know you. Therefore, you must greet, introduce yourself and incorporate any necessary courtesies before asking diagnostic questions. If necessary, review information from previous chapters regarding proper courtesy. After completing all of the situations, switch roles.

Patient:	Find Out:
1. Sr. Quiñones (kee-**nyoh**-nays)	• if he's had fried, greasy foods • how often he eats such food • if he is constipated or has had cramps • if he drinks alcohol or coffee • if there has been blood in his stool
2. Srta. Saucedo (sah^oo-**say**-doh)	• if some foods disagree with her • if she has heartburn or diarrhea • how often and when it occurs • if she drinks sodas or whole milk
3. Sra. Alvarez (**ahl**-bah-rays)	• how often she suffers from gas • if she drinks beer, wine or other alcoholic beverages • if she eats red meat, white meat, fish or seafood • if it hurts to have a bowel movement
4. Sr. Villanueva (bee-yah-**noo**^ay-bah)	• if he eats late at night • if he eats vegetables, breads and cereals • if certain foods don't agree with him • if he has cramps or if it hurts to defecate

B) Matching

Instructions: Match the beginning of each phrase with its proper ending. Then, translate them into ENGLISH. Check your answers only when you have finished.

1. ___ ¿Toma el . . .	a. mucho?
2. ___ ¿Toma comidas . . .	b. le caigan mal?
3. ___ ¿Con qué frecuencia . . .	c. leche desnatada?
4. ___ ¿Come muy . . .	d. todos los días?
5. ___ ¿Toma . . .	e. desayuno regularmente?
6. ___ ¿Eructa . . .	f. grasosas o fritas?
7. ___ ¿Va de vientre . . .	g. toma agua?
8. ___ ¿Hay comidas que . . .	h. tarde por la noche?

Section VI
Musculoskelatal System

Before You Begin

Since the average person's knowledge of human anatomy is limited, regardless of ethnicity, a patient's description of where he or she feels pain may be difficult to interpret. You may encounter Hispanic patients that will use the word *el cerebro (ayl say-ray-broh)*, literally *brain*, to describe the location of a headache that starts at the back of the head and radiates down the neck. Likewise, some patients may refer to the location of upper paraspinal musculoskeletal pain as being in *el pulmón (ayl pool-mohn)*. This is actually the singular word for *lung*. Commonly, many Hispanics will also complain of *kidney pain (dolor en los riñones / doh-lohr ayn lohs rree-nyoh-nays)* or *waist pain (dolor en la cintura / doh-lohr ayn lah seen-too-rah)* when experiencing lower back pain.

Phrases

English	Pronunciation & Spanish
1. Do your . . . ache?	*lay **dway**-layn . . .* ¿Le duelen . . . [1]
joints	*lahs ahr-tee-koo-lah-**see^oh**-nays?* las articulaciones?
muscles	*lohs **moo**-skoo-lohs?* los músculos
bones	*lohs **way**-sohs?* los huesos?
2. Does your . . . ache?	*lay **dway**-lay . . .* ¿Le duele . . . [1]
(upper/lower) back	*lah ay-**spahl**-dah (soo-pay-**ree^ohr** / een-fay-**ree^ohr**)?* la espalda (superior / inferior)?
neck	*ayl **kway**-yoh?* el cuello?
3. Does the pain radiate out?	*say **koh**-rray ayl doh-**lohr**?* ¿Se corre el dolor?
4. Will you point out for me	*may say-**nyah**-lah kohn ayl **day**-doh* ¿Me señala con el dedo
where the pain begins?	***dohn**-day koh-**mee^ayn**-sah ayl doh-**lohr**?* dónde comienza el dolor?
5. Will you trace with your finger the path	*may **trah**-sah kohn ayl **day**-doh ayl trah^ee-**yayk**-toh* ¿Me traza con el dedo el trayecto
of the pain to where it radiates out?	*dayl doh-**lohr** ah-stah **dohn**-day say ayk-**stee^ayn**-day?* del dolor hasta dónde se extiende? [2]
6. How often do you have pain?	*kohn kay fray-**kwayn**-see^ah **tee^ay**-nay doh-**lohr**?* ¿Con qué frecuencia tiene dolor? [3]

7. Do you have . . .

tee^ay-nay . . .
¿Tiene . . .

    muscle weakness?

*day-bee-lee-**dahd** moo-skoo-**lahr?***
debilidad muscular?

    tingling in some area?

*ohr-mee-**gay**-ohs ayn ahl-**goon** loo-**gahr?***
hormigueos en algún lugar?

    (involuntary) spasms?

*ay-**spahs**-mohs (een-voh-loon-**tah**-ree^ohs)?*
espasmos (involuntarios)?

    numbness in some area?

*ayn-too-may-see-**mee^ayn**-toh ayn ahl-**goon** loo-**gahr?***
entumecimiento en algún lugar?

8. Have you ever had a . . .

*ah tay-**nee**-doh ahl-**goo**-nah bays . . .*
¿Ha tenido alguna vez . . .

    fracture?

*frak-**too**-rah?*
fractura?

    broken bone?

***way**-soh **rroh**-toh?*
hueso roto?

    dislocation?

*look-sah-**see^ohn?***
luxación?[4]

    swelling on a bone?

*een-chay-**sohn** ayn ahl-**goon** **way**-soh?*
hinchazón en algún hueso?

9. Will you show me where?

*may say-**nyah**-lah **dohn**-day?*
¿Me señala dónde?

Notes

[1] Use the *PAIN SCALE* found in **APPENDIX: Chapter 9 - Assessing the Patient's Problem - Preliminary Questions/Pain Assessment** to help in assessing the severity of discomfort.

[2] Since you are speaking of back/neck pain, you may want to use the *BODY DIAGRAMS* in the **APPENDIX** to allow patients to answer this question. They may simply indicate on the diagram the point of origin and path of pain radiation by tracing it for you.

[3] Use the *FREQUENCY CHART* found in **APPENDIX: Chapter 9 - Assessing the Patient's Problem - Cardiopulmonary System.**

[4] Also, the cognate *dislocación (dees-loh-kah-see^ohn)* is commonly heard.

Practical Activities VI

A) Oral Practice

Instructions: In pairs, one person will play the role of the health care provider and the other will play the role of the patient. Whomever is playing the patient will imagine beforehand the location of a pain without revealing it to the person playing the health care provider. The objective of the health care provider is to obtain information from the patient using SPANISH only and then write notes in ENGLISH about what (s)he finds out in the patient's chart (on a scratch sheet of paper). Of course, the patient will respond only in SPANISH, using body language and hand gestures as well. Make sure to incorporate the *PAIN SCALE, FREQUENCY CHART* and *BODY DIAGRAMS* to facilitate communication. After completing the patient's assessment, switch roles and recreate the situation.

The health care provider will find out . . .

- if any joints, muscles or bones ache.
- if the neck or back aches.
- if the pain radiates and if so, from where to where.
- how often the pain occurs.
- what the pain feels like.
  (Use questions from Chapter 9: Preliminary Questions/Pain Assessment.)
- if there are any additional symptoms, such as tingling, spasms, etc. and where.
- if the patient has ever broken or fractured a bone and if so, where.
- if the patient has ever dislocated a joint and if so, where.

B) Matching

Instructions: Using the *Body Diagrams* from the Appendix for **Chapter 9**, match the SPANISH body part with the ENGLISH meaning. Then go to **Chapter 17: Parts of the Body** and practice saying each one in SPANISH.

The Human Body — Rear View / El cuerpo humano — vista posterior

1. ___ head	a. hombro		8. ___ buttock	h. cadera
2. ___ nape	b. cóccix		9. ___ back	i. mano
3. ___ armpit	c. nalga		10. ___ hip	j. talón
4. ___ shoulder	d. cabeza		11. ___ hamstring	k. axila
5. ___ forearm	e. espalda		12. ___ calf	l. recto
6. ___ coccyx	f. pantorilla		13. ___ heel	m. antebrazo
7. ___ hand	g. nuca		14. ___ rectum	n. posterior del muslo

Section VII
Neurological System

Phrases

English	Pronunciation & Spanish
1. Do you have . . .	*tee^ay-nay . . .* ¿Tiene . . .
tingling in some area?	*ohr-mee-**gay**-ohs ayn ahl-**goon** loo-**gahr**?* hormigueos en algún lugar?
numbness in some area?	*ayn-too-may-see-**mee^ayn**-toh ayn ahl-**goon** loo-**gahr**?* entumecimiento en algún lugar?
vertigo?	***bayr**-tee-goh?* vértigo?
a good memory?	***bway**-nah may-**moh**-ree^ah?* buena memoria?
good balance?	*bwayn ay-kee-**lee**-bree^oh?* buen equilibrio?
2. Will you show me where?	*may say-**nyah**-lah **dohn**-day?* ¿Me señala dónde?[1]
3. How often do you have	*kohn kay fray-**kwayn**-see^ah **tee^ay**-nay* ¿Con qué frecuencia tiene
those sensations/problems?	***tah**-lays sayn-sah-**see^oh**-nays / proh-**blay**-mahs?* tales sensaciones / problemas?[2]
4. Is your . . .	*ays soo . . .* ¿Es su . . .
memory . . .	*may-**moh**-ree^ah . . .* memoria . . .
balance . . .	*ay-kee-**lee**-bree^oh . . .* equilibrio . . .
worse than before?	*pay-**ohr** kay **ahn**-tays?* peor que antes?
same as before?	*ee-**gwahl** kay **ahn**-tays?* igual que antes?
5. Is it difficult for you . . .	*lay ays dee-**fee**-seel . . .* ¿Le es difícil . . .
to walk?	*kah-mee-**nahr**?* caminar?
move?	*moh-**bayr**-say?* moverse?

keep your balance?	*mahn-tay-**nayr** ayl ay-kee-**lee**-bree^oh?* mantener el equilibrio?
distinguish between hot	*dee-steen-**gheer ayn**-tray ayl kah-**lohr*** distinguir entre el calor
and cold on you skin?	*ee ayl **free**-oh ayn lah pee^ayl?* y el frío en la piel?

6. Have you ever lost your sense of touch?	*ah payr-**dee**-doh ahl-**goo**-nah bays lah sayn-see-bee-lee-**dahd tahk**-teel?* ¿Ha perdido alguna vez la sensibilidad táctil?

7. Have you noticed a change in	*ah noh-**tah**-doh oon **kahm**-bee^oh ayn ayl* ¿Ha notado un cambio en el
the way a particular food tastes?	*sah-**bohr** day ahl-**goo**-nah koh-**mee**-dah ayn pahr-tee-koo-**lahr**?* sabor de alguna comida en particular?

Notes

[1] Since you are speaking of specific locations on the body, you may want to use the *BODY DIAGRAMS* in the **APPENDIX** to allow patients to answer this question. They may simply indicate on the diagram the origin by pointing it out for you.

[2] Use the *FREQUENCY CHART* found in **APPENDIX: Chapter 9 - Assessing the Patient's Problem - Diagnostic Questions - Cardiopulmonary System.**

Practical Activities VII

A) Oral Practice

Instructions: Read the following notes from a Spanish-speaking patient's chart. Then, look for general information that would need more detail. Lastly, prepare 6 to 8 different follow-up questions in SPANISH that you would ask the patient to obtain these necessary details. You may want to include the charts and diagrams from the appendix for Chapter 9 to assist you. After you have prepared your follow-up questions, find a partner and prepare the conversation in SPANISH between health care provider and patient. Remember to take turns, allowing each person to play both roles.

Notes from patient chart:

10/15/2006 -
Patient complains of tingling sensations and experiences temporary bouts of localized numbness. He (She) also finds it difficult to walk due to problems with balance and dizziness. The patient has also mentioned changes in tactile perception and says some food and drink have a slightly metallic aftertaste.

Example:

You read in the patient's chart that (s)he *complains of tingling sensations*. You would want to follow-up with questions or requests such as *Can you show me where?, How often?, etc.*, but in SPANISH, of course.

B) Patient Chart Update

Instructions: You have just read the notes from a patient's chart and asked your own follow-up questions to ascertain more detailed information. Now, you are going to make your own notes in the patient's chart based on his/her responses. Since you have rehearsed the health care provider/patient conversation, repeat it once more, uninterrupted, and record the patient responses in ENGLISH below as you and the patient converse in SPANISH. After you are done, switch roles and allow your partner to do the same thing. Compare your notes after you have both written them down to check the written notes against the patient's verbal responses.

Section VIII
Male and Female Genitourinary System/STDs

Before You Begin

It is very common for Hispanic females to feel uneasy speaking with a medical professional, especially a male, about sexual issues. Their reluctance may be attributed to a patient's education level and/or cultural taboos. Remember to approach such topics sensitively.

The attitudes adopted by Hispanics regarding contraceptives and reproduction are directly influenced by cultural and religious beliefs as well as the level of education and socioeconomic status. Even a male not wanting his wife to become pregnant will often insist that she not use any type of contraceptive, since the belief that a woman herself is responsible for birth control is still a widely accepted misconception. Many times, the disdain for contraceptives can be traced to deep-rooted Roman Catholic beliefs and teachings that the majority of Hispanics traditionally follow.

The Hispanic population finds itself at an increased risk for HIV not because of race or culture but due to such components as living in areas where there is a greater risk of exposure to IV drug use. Heterosexual transmission of HIV between an IV drug user and partner is more common than one would expect due to the cultural atttitude toward the use of condoms (contraceptives).

HIV exposure for Hispanic men occurs primarily through homosexual encounters, whereas the majority of Hispanic women are exposed through heterosexual sex. However, Hispanics are more likely to get tested for HIV than any other ethnic group.

Hispanics in the U.S. are disproportionately affected by STDs. There are many complex issues regarding sexuality, gender, faith and immigration that count as contributing factors to the elevated infection rates. Other contributors include, language barriers, legal status, clinic hours, cultural differences, lack of health insurance and insufficient transportation.

Phrases

English	Pronunciation & Spanish
1. Do you have problems urinating?	*tee^**ay**-nay proh-**blay**-mahs ahl oh-ree-**nahr**?* ¿Tiene problemas al orinar?
2. Do have the urge to urinate frequently?	*tee^**ay**-nay oor-**hayn**-see^ah day oh-ree-**nahr** kohn fray-**kwayn**-see^ah?* ¿Tiene urgencia de orinar con frecuencia?
3. How often do you urinate?	*kohn kay fray-**kwayn**-see^ah oh-**ree**-nah?* ¿Con qué frecuencia orina?[1]
4. Do you get up at night to urinate?	*say lay-**bahn**-tah pohr lah **noh**-chay **pah**-rah oh-ree-**nahr**?* ¿Se levanta por la noche para orinar?
5. Do you now have or have you had	*tee^**ay**-nay ah-**oh**-rah oh ah tay-**nee**-doh* ¿Tiene ahora o ha tenido
pain in . . .	*doh-**lohr** day . . .* dolor de . . . [2]
your kidneys?	*lohs rree-**nyoh**-nays?* los riñones?
your bladder?	*lah bay-**hee**-gah?* la vejiga?

6. Does it hurt to urinate?

*tee^ay-nay doh-**lohr** ahl oh-ree-**nahr**?*
¿Tiene dolor al orinar?

7. Does it hurt to . . . urinating?

*tee^ay-nay doh-**lohr** ahl . . . oh-ree-**nahr**?*
¿Tiene dolor al . . . orinar?

start

*koh-mayn-**sahr** ah*
comenzar a

stop

*tayr-may-**nahr** day*
terminar de

8. Have you had . . .

*ah tay-**nee**-doh . . .*
¿Ha tenido . . .

kidney stones?

*kahl-koo-lohs ayn lohs rree-**nyoh**-nays?*
cálculos en los riñones?

small stones in your urine?

*ah-ray-**nee**-yah ayn lah oh-**ree**-nah?*
arenilla en la orina?

stones in your urine?

*pee^ay-drahs ayn lah oh-**ree**-nah?*
piedras en la orina?

a kidney infection?

*oo-nah een-fayk-**see^ohn** day rree-**nyoh**-nays?*
una infección de riñones?

a bladder infection?

*oo-nah een-fayk-**see^ohn** day bay-**hee**-gah?*
una infección de vejiga?

9. Have you noticed . . . in your urine?

*ah noh-**tah**-doh . . . ayn lah oh-**ree**-nah?*
¿Ha notado . . . en la orina?

blood

sahn-gray
sangre

pus

poos
pus

10. Is your urine . . .

*ays lah oh-**ree**-nah . . .*
¿Es la orina . . .

clear?

klah-rah?
clara?

yellow?

*ah-mah-**ree**-yah?*
amarilla?

cloudy?

toor-bee^ah?
turbia?

milky?

*lay-**choh**-sah?*
lechosa?

reddish?

*rroh-**hee**-sah?*
rojiza?

11. Do you have now or have you had . . .

*tee^ay-nay ah-**oh**-rah oh ah tay-**nee**-doh . . .*
¿Tiene ahora o ha tenido . . .

prostate problems?	*proh-**blay**-mahs day lah **proh**-stah-tah?* problemas de la próstata?
an inflamed prostate?	*lah **proh**-stah-tah een-flah-**mah**-dah?* la próstata inflamada?
sores on your penis?	***ool**-say-rahs ayn lah **pay**-nay?* úlceras en el pene?
12. When was your last period?	***kwahn**-doh fway soo **ool**-tee-mah mayn-stroo^ah-**see**^ohn?* ¿Cuándo fue su última menstruación? [4]
13. Are you on your period now?	*lah **tee**^ay-nay ah-**oh**-rah?* ¿La tiene ahora?
14. How often do you get your period?	*kohn kay fray-**kwayn**-see^ah **tee**^ay-nay soo mayn-stroo^ah-**see**^ohn?* ¿Con qué frecuencia tiene su menstruación? [1]
15. How many days does it last?	*pohr **kwahn**-tohs **dee**-ahs **doo**-rah?* ¿Por cuántos días dura? [1]
16. Do you bleed a lot or a little?	*lay **sah**-lay **moo**-chah oh **poh**-kah **sahn**-gray?* ¿Le sale mucha o poca sangre?
17. Have your periods been regular?	*ahn **see**-doh rray-goo-**lah**-rays soos mayn-stroo^ah-**see**^oh-nays?* ¿Han sido regulares sus menstruaciones?
18. Do you have pain with your period?	***tee**^ay-nay doh-**lohr** kohn lah mayn-stroo^ah-**see**^ohn?* ¿Tiene dolor con la menstruación?
19. Do you suffer from severe	***soo**-fray day kah-**lahm**-brays* ¿Sufre de calambres
menstrual cramping?	*mayn-**stroo^ah**-lays say-**bay**-rohs?* menstruales severos?
20. Have you suffered any	*ah soo-**free**-doh day ahl-**goon*** ¿Ha sufrido de algún
menstrual problems?	*trah-**stohr**-noh mayn-**stroo^ahl**?* trastorno menstrual?
21. Are you pregnant?	*ay-**stah** aym-bah-rah-**sah**-dah?* ¿Está embarazada?
22. Have you been pregnant?	*ah ay-**stah**-doh aym-bah-rah-**sah**-dah?* ¿Ha estado embarazada?
23. How many times?	***kwahn**-tahs **bay**-says?* ¿Cuántas veces? [1]
24. Was the birth . . .	*fway ayl **pahr**-toh . . .* ¿Fue el parto . . .
normal?	*nohr-**mahl**?* normal?
induced?	*een-doo-**see**-doh?* inducido?

	*pohr oh-pay-rah-**see**^**ohn** say-**sah**-ree-ah?*
by Cesarean section?	¿por operación cesárea?

---

	*ah tay-**nee**-doh ahl-**goo**-nah bays . . .*
25. Have you ever had . . .	¿Ha tenido alguna vez . . .
	*mahl-**pahr**-toh?*
a miscarriage?	malparto?
	*ah-**bohr**-toh (een-doo-**see**-doh / ay-spohn-**tah**-nay-oh)?*
an (induced/spontaneous) abortion?	aborto (inducido / espontáneo)?

---

	*oo-sah ahn-tee-kohn-sayp-**tee**-bohs?*
26. Do you use contraceptives?	¿Usa anticonceptivos?

---

	*ay-**stah** sah-tees-**fay**-choh/chah kohn soo **bee**-dah sayk-**soo**^**ahl**?*
27. Are you happy with your sex life?	¿Está satisfecho/a con su vida sexual? [5]

---

	*ah tay-**nee**-doh **oo**-nah ayn-fayr-may-**dahd***
28. Have you ever had a sexually	¿Ha tenido una enfermedad
	*trahns-mee-**tee**-dah sayk-soo^ahl-**mayn**-tay?*
transmitted disease?	transmitida sexualmente?

---

	kwahl fway?
29. What was it?	¿Cuál fue? [3]

---

	*ay-**stah** seer-koon-**see**-soh?*
30. Are you circumcised?	¿Está circunciso?

---

	*ay-**stah** seer-koon-**see**-sah soo pah-**ray**-hah?*
31. Is your partner circumcised?	¿Está circuncisa su pareja?

---

	*ah noh-**tah**-doh . . .*
32. Have you noticed . . .	¿Ha notado . . .
	*doh-**lohr** . . .*
pain . . .	dolor . . .
	*een-chah-**sohn** . . .*
swelling . . .	hinchazón . . .
	*boh-**lee**-tah(s) . . .*
a lump(s) . . .	bolita(s) . . .
	*ayn lohs **sat**-nohs?*
in your breasts?	en los senos?
	*ayn lohs tay-**stee**-koo-lohs?*
in your testicles?	en los testículos?

---

	*ah noh-**tah**-doh ahl-**goo**-nah say-kray-**see**^**ohn** . . .*
33. Have you noticed any discharge from . . .	¿Ha notado alguna secreción . . .
	*day lohs **say**-nohs?*
your breasts?	de los senos?
	*day lah bah-**hee**-nah?*
your vagina?	de la vagina?

your penis?	*dayl **pay**-nay?* del pene?

---

34. Do you have any . . .	***tee^ay**-nay . . .* ¿Tiene . . . ?
itching . . .	*pee-kah-**sohn** . . .* picazón . . .
redness . . .	*ayn-roh-hay-see-**mee^ayn**-toh . . .* enrojecimiento . . .
burning sensation . . .	*ahr-**dohr** . . .* ardor . . .
rash . . .	*sahl-poo-**yee**-doh . . .* salpullido . . .
in your genital region?	*ayn lohs hay-nay-**tah**-lays?* en los genitales?
on another part of your body?	*ayn **oh**-trah **pahr**-tay dayl **kwayr**-poh?* en otra parte del cuerpo?

---

35. Have you had these symptoms	***ah**-say **moo**-choh oh **poh**-koh **tee^aym**-poh* ¿Hace mucho o poco tiempo
for a long or short period of time?	*kay **tee^ay**-nay **ay**-stohs **seen**-toh-mahs?* que tiene estos síntomas?

---

36. Have you had sexual relations	*ah tay-**nee**-doh rray-lah-**see^oh**-nays sayk-**soo^ah**-lays* ¿Ha tenido relaciones sexuales
recently?	*rray-see^ayn-tay-**mayn**-tay?* recientemente?

---

37. Do you know if your partner	***sah**-bay see soo pah-**ray**-hah **tee^ay**-nay* ¿Sabe si su pareja tiene
has the same symptoms?	*lohs **mees**-mohs **seen**-toh-mahs?* los mismos síntomas?

---

38. Do you practice safe sex?	*prahk-**tee**-kah ayl **sayk**-soh say-**goo**-roh?* ¿Practica el sexo seguro?

---

39. You need to go to an STD clinic.	*nay-say-**see**-tah eer ah **oo**-nah **klee**-nee-kah* Necesita ir a una clínica
	*day ayn-fayr-may-**dah**-days trahns-mee-**tee**-dahs sayk-soo^ahl-**mayn**-tay.* de enfermedades transmitidas sexualmente.

---

40. We can give you a referral.	*lay poh-**day**-mohs dahr **oo**-nah rray-koh-mayn-dah-**see^ohn**.* Le podemos dar una recomendación.

---

41. For now, you shouldn't . . .	*pohr ah-**oh**-rah noh **day**-bay . . .* Por ahora, no debe . . .
have sexual relations.	*tay-**nayr** rray-lah-**see^oh**-nays sayk-**soo^ah**-lays.* tener relaciones sexuales.

drink alcohol.	*bay-**bayr** ahl-koh-**ohl**.* beber alcohol.
do physical exercise.	*ah-**sayr** ay-hayr-**see**-see^oh **fee**-see-koh.* hacer ejercicio físico.

Notes

[1] Use the *FREQUENCY CHART* found in **APPENDIX: Chapter 9 - Assessing the Patient's Problem - Diagnostic Questions - Cardiopulmonary System.**

[2] Remember you can always go back to **APPENDIX: Chapter 9 - Assessing the Patient's Problem - Preliminary Questions/Pain Assessment** to help in assessing the severity of discomfort and use the accompanying *PAIN SCALE.*

[3] If possible, have the patient write this information for you. Many of these terms are *cognates*, meaning they look a lot like the English word and are fairly easy to recognize.

[4] Using the cards from **APPENDIX: Chapter 2 - General Administration - Making Appointments and Scheduling Follow-up Visits** lay the name of the month and the days of the week over those of your desk calendar. Now you have a bilingual visual reference.

[5] Use *satisfecho* with a *male patient* and *satisfecha* with a *female patient.*

Practical Activities VIII

A) Oral Practice

Instructions: Imagine you are about to see your first patient of the day. In pairs, assign the role of patient and the role of health care provider. Then, using the cues below, ask the patient the appropriate questions to obtain the information indicated speaking only in SPANISH. Record his/her answers in English on the table below. Remember, you may need to use charts and/or diagrams from the appendix for this chapter. Once you are done, switch roles and recreate the situation. Practice both female and male patient questions.

female patient cues	response	male patient cues	response
1. problems urinating		1. prostate problems	
2. frequent urination		2. STDs	
3. pain in kidneys		3. satisfying sex life	
4. painful urination		4. circumcised	
5. blood in urine		5. genital redness	
6. last period		6. duration of symptoms	
7. duration of period		7. recent sexual relations	
8. severe cramping		8. safe sex	

B) ¿Hombre o mujer?

Instructions: The following table contains a variety of questions from this section. Read each one, then decide if the question would be appropriate for a *male*, a *female* or *both*. Indicate your response by writing the letters *m* for *male*, *f* for *female* or *b* for *both*. After you have finished, check your responses with the English phrases from this section.

m/f/b	Questions	m/f/b	Questions
_____	1. ¿Ha notado alguna secreción de los senos?	_____	6. ¿Usa anticonceptivos?
_____	2. ¿Se levanta por la noche para orinar?	_____	7. ¿Ha notado hinchazón en los testículos?
_____	3. ¿Tiene dolor al terminar de orinar?	_____	8. ¿Tiene enrojecimiento en otra parte del cuerpo?
_____	4. ¿Tiene ahora úlceras en el pene?	_____	9. ¿Hace mucho o poco tiempo que tiene estos síntomas?
_____	5. ¿Está embarazada?	_____	10. ¿Practica el sexo seguro?

Cyber-Investigation

As you learned in **Before You Begin** at the beginning of this chapter, males play a very dominant role in the Hispanic family. This is embodied in the concept of *machismo*. Do an Internet search for this term and find 3 to 4 different ways in which *machismo* may directly impact not only a male Hispanic and his views on health care but also those of his wife and family. Share this information with your class.

Chapter 10

Laboratory Examinations and Procedures

Section I
Patient Instructions Prior to Procedure

Before You Begin

It is important to note that, due to the invasive nature of some procedures, the extreme modesty of Hispanic women, and traditional cultural norms that are quite prevalent among Hispanics, the health care professional should be the same sex as the patient.

Since modesty is extremely important for Hispanic females, they should be provided with as much privacy as possible for any medical procedure. Studies have shown that Hispanic females are also less likely to perform self-examination of their breasts or get Pap smears, due to sexual associations of these examinations. The later directly contributes to a high rate of cervical cancer.

Phrases

English	Pronunciation & Spanish
1. We need to schedule you for . . .	*nay-say-see-**tah**-mohs proh-grah-**mahr**-lay **oo**-nah **see**-tah **pah**-rah . . .* Necesitamos programarle una cita para . . .
an X-ray.	***oo**-nah rrah-dee^oh-grah-**fee**-ah* una radiografía.[1]
a blood test.	*oon ah-**nah**-lee-sees day **sahn**-gray* un análisis de sangre.
a throat culture.	*oon kool-**tee**-boh day gahr-**gahn**-tah.* un cultivo de garganta.
a stool culture.	*oon kool-**tee**-boh day ayk-skray-**mayn**-toh.* un cultivo de excremento.
a urine test.	***oo**-nah **proo^ay**-bah day oh-**ree**-nah.* una prueba de orina.
a mammogram.	*oon mah-moh-**grah**-mah.* un mamograma.
a scan.	*oon ay-**skahn**.* un escán.[1]

119

some tests.	*ah-**sayr**-lay **oo**-nohs ah-**nah**-lee-sees.* hacerle unos análisis.
2. I am going to give you instructions on	*lay boy ah dahr een-strook-**see^oh**-nays day* Le voy a dar instrucciones de
what you need to do	*loh kay **day**-bay day ah-**sayr*** lo que debe de hacer
before your procedure.	***ahn**-tays day soo proh-say-dee-**mee^ayn**-toh.* antes de su procedimiento.
3. You will need to fast	*nay-say-**see**-tah ay-**stahr** day ah^ee-**oo**-nahs* Necesita estar de ayunas
before the procedure.	***ahn**-tays dayl proh-say-dee-**mee^ayn**-toh.* antes del procedimiento.
4. Begin . . .	*aym-**pee^ay**-say . . .* Empiece . . .
at midnight . . .	*lah may-dee^ah-**noh**-chay . . .* la medianoche . . .
the night . . .	*la **noh**-chay . . .* la noche . . .
two hours . . .	*dohs **oh**-rahs . . .* dos horas . . .
three hours . . .	*trays **oh**-rahs . . .* tres horas . . .
twelve hours . . .	***doh**-say **oh**-rahs . . .* doce horas . . .
before your appointment for	***ahn**-tays day soo **see**-tah **pah**-rah* antes de su cita para
the procedure.	*ayl proh-say-dee-**mee^ayn**-toh.* el procedimiento.
5. It is important not to . . . before	*ays eem-pohr-**tahn**-tay noh . . . **ahn**-tays dayl* Es importante no . . . antes del
the procedure.	*proh-say-dee-**mee^ayn**-toh.* procedimiento.
eat	*koh-**mayr*** comer
drink (nothing but water)	*bay-**bayr** (**nah**-dah **sahl**-boh **ah**-gwah)* beber (nada salvo agua)
chew gum	*mahs-tee-**kahr** **chee**-klay* masticar chicle

smoke	*foo-**mahr*** fumar	
take medicine	*toh-**mahr** may-dee-**see**-nah* tomar medicina	
put anything in your mouth	*poh-**nayr nah**-dah ayn lah **boh**-kah* poner nada en la boca	

6. Before your procedure you must . . .

    *ahn-tays dayl proh-say-dee-**mee^ayn**-toh **day**-bay day . . .*
    Antes del procedimiento, debe de . . .

    eat something light.

    *toh-**mahr** oo-nah koh-**mee**-dah lee-**hay**-rah.*
    tomar una comida ligera.

    eat a hearty meal.

    *toh-**mahr** oo-nah koh-**mee**-dah soo-stahn-**see^ahl**.*
    tomar una comida sustancial.

    take these pills.

    *toh-**mahr** ay-stahs pah-**stee**-yahs.*
    tomar estas pastillas.

    drink this liquid.

    *toh-**mahr** ay-stay **lee**-kee-doh.*
    tomar este líquido.

7. If you don't follow these instructions

    *see noh **see**-gay lahs een-strook-**see^oh**-nays*
    Si no sigue las instrucciones

    carefully, they will not be able

    *ah-tayn-tah-**mayn**-tay noh poh-**drahn***
    atentamente, no podrán

    to perform the procedure and you will

    *ah-**sayr**-lay ayl proh-say-dee-**mee^ayn**-toh ee tayn-**drah** kay*
    hacerle el procedimiento y tendrá que

    have to reschedule.

    *rray-proh-grah-**mahr** lah **see**-tah.*
    reprogramar la cita.

8. This is the form you will need

    *ay-stay ays ayl fohr-moo-**lah**-ree^oh kay **day**-bay*
    Este es el formulario que debe

    to give to the lab tech.

    *day **dahr**-lay ahl **tayk**-nee-koh.*
    de darle al técnico.

9. This form contains the doctor's

    *ay-stay fohr-moo-**lah**-ree^oh kohn-**tee^ay**-nay lahs*
    Este formulario contiene las

    written orders.

    *een-dee-kah-**see^oh**-nays ay-**skree**-tahs dayl dohk-**tohr** / day lah dohk-**toh**-rah.*
    indicaciones escritas del doctor / de la doctora.[2]

Notes

[1] Since there are numerous reasons for x-rays and scans, you may choose to indicate *of what* by using *de (day)* + *the organ/body part* from Chapter 17. For example, "a scan of the gall bladder" would be "un escán de la vesícula biliar".

[2] Use *del doctor* if you are speaking of a male doctor and *de la doctora* if you are speaking of a female doctor. If the gender is unknown use *del doctor*.

Practical Activities I

A) Oral Practice

Instructions: You are telling two different patients they have been scheduled for a laboratory procedure. According to the information given in the table below, prepare what you will say to each patient in SPANISH. Do not repeat dialogue used for PATIENT #1 in the dialogue you prepare for PATIENT #2 when possible. Also, remember this is not a conversation but rather straightforward information. After you have prepared your dialogue, form groups of 3 to 4 and practice giving your information as if one of the group's members were your patient. The other members of the group should make notes in ENGLISH to test their own comprehension of the instructions.

Tell Patient #1:

- which procedure he will have
- you are going to give him instructions
- to start fasting the night before
- not to (choose 2 items from #3 this section)
- not to put anything in his mouth
- to give this form to the lab tech

Tell Patient #2:

- which procedure she will have
- you are going to give her instructions
- to drink this liquid and take these pills
- to eat something light beforehand
- to follow the instructions thoroughly
- this form contains the doctor's instructions

B) Doctor's Written Orders

Instructions: Translate the doctor's written orders from SPANISH to ENGLISH in the space provided below. Try not to refer back to the chapter until you are finished, then, check your translation. Compare your translation with a classmate before referring back to the phrases in this section.

Necesitamos programarle una cita para un cultivo de excremento. Le voy a dar instrucciones de lo que debe de hacer antes de su procedimiento. Necesita estar de ayunas antes de su procedimiento. Empiece tres horas antes. Es importante no comer ni ("nor") beber nada salvo agua antes del procedimiento. Si no sigue las instrucciones, no podrán hacerle el procedimiento y tendrá que reprogramar la cita. Este es el formulario que debe de darle al técnico.

Section II
Laboratory Examinations and Procedures: The X-Ray

Phrases

English	Pronunciation & Spanish
1. I'm the lab tech.	*soy ayl tayk-nee-koh / lah tayk-nee-kah.* Soy el técnico / la técnica.[1]
2. Do you have the orders from your doctor?	*tee^ay-nay lahs een-dee-kah-see^oh-nays ay-skree-tahs day soo dohk-tohr?* ¿Tiene las indicaciones escritas de su doctor?
3. Did you follow the doctor's orders exactly as indicated?	*see-ghee-oh lahs een-dee-kah-see^oh-nays* ¿Siguió las indicaciones *ay-skree-tahs ah-tayn-tah-mayn-tay?* escritas atentamente?
4. If not, I will not be able to do the procedure.	*see kay noh noh poh-dray ah-sayr-lay* Si que no, no podré hacerle *ayl proh-say-dee-mee^ayn-toh.* el procedimiento.
5. Take off your clothes and put this on, please.	*days-bee-stay-say ee pon-gah-say ay-stoh* Desvístese y póngase esto, *pohr fah-bohr.* por favor.[2]
6. Stand here with your arms by your side.	*pon-gah-say ah-kee kohn lohs brah-sohs ah lohs koh-stah-dohs.* Póngase aquí con los brazos a los costados.[3]
7. Lie down on the table with your arms by your side, please.	*ah-kway-stay-say ayn lah may-sah kohn lohs brah-sohs* Acúestese en la mesa con los brazos *ah lohs koh-stah-dohs pohr fah-bohr.* a los costados, por favor.
8. Allow me to position you. Relax your body.	*payr-mee-tah-may poh-nayr-lay ayn lah poh-stoo-rah koh-rrayk-tah.* Permítame ponerle en la postura correcta. *rray-lah-hay ayl kwayr-poh.* Relaje el cuerpo.[4]
9. Hold this position until I tell you to relax.	*ah-gwahn-tay lah poh-stoo-rah ah-stah* Aguante la postura hasta *kay lay dee-gah kay say rray-lah-hay.* que le diga que se relaje.
10. Good.	*bee^ayn.* Bien.[5]
11. Hold it.	*ah-gwahn-tay-lah.* Aguántela.[5]

12. Don't move.	*noh say **mway**-bah.* No se mueva.[5]
13. Now, take a deep breath.	*ah-**oh**-rah **toh**-may oon rray-**spee**-roh **ohn**-doh.* Ahora, tome un respiro hondo.[5]
14. Hold it.	*ah-**gwahn**-tay-loh.* Aguántelo.[5]
15. Don't breathe.	*noh rray-**spee**-ray.* No respire.[5]
16. Breathe.	*rray-**spee**-ray.* Respire.[5]
17. I am going to take the x-ray now.	*boy ah toh-**mahr**-lay lah rrah-dee^oh-grah-**fee**-ah ah-**oh**-rah.* Voy a tomarle la radiografía ahora.[5]
18. I need to repeat this process	*nay-say-**see**-toh rray-pay-**teer** ayl proh-**say**-soh* Necesito repetir el proceso
one more time.	***oo**-nah bays mahs.* una vez más.
19. I need to repeat this	*nay-say-**see**-toh rray-pay-**teer** ayl* Necesito repetir el
process . . . more times.	*proh-**say**-soh . . . bay-**says mahs.*** proceso . . . veces más.
two	*dohs* dos
three	*trays* tres
four	***kwah**-troh* cuatro
five	***seen**-koh* cinco
20. Wait a moment, I need to see	*ay-**spay**-ray oon moh-**mayn**-toh nay-say-**see**-toh bayr* Espere un momento, necesito ver
if the x-ray(s) turned out okay.	*see ah(n) sah-**lee**-doh bee^ayn lah(s) rrah-dee^oh-grah-**fee**-ah(s).* si ha(n) salido bien la(s) radiografía(s).
21. Thank you, we're done.	***grah**-see^ahs **ay**-mohs tayr-mee-**nah**-doh.* Gracias, hemos terminado.
22. Someone will call you with the results.	***ahl**-ghee^ayn lay yah-mah-**rah** kohn lohs rray-sool-**tah**-dohs.* Alguien le llamará con los resultados.

Notes

[1] Use *el técnico* if you are male and *la técnica* if you are female.

[2] Remember, using gestures and body language will facilitate communication with these types of expressions.

[3] Point to where you would like the patient to stand.

[4] Use this phrase in lieu of having to remember many commands to have the patient position him/herself. As always, say it but wait a moment until the patient indicates (s)he is comfortable with you positioning him/her.

[5] Repeat these phrases liberally to assist you in the process of taking an x-ray. Feel free to manipulate order to best suit your needs.

Practical Activities II

A) Oral Practice

Instructions: You are taking X-rays of a patient per the written orders of his/her doctor. The patient speaks no ENGLISH and is unfamiliar with the process. Instruct the patient step-by-step as to what (s)he needs to do using a miniumum of 10 expressions from this section. After you have prepared your instructions, have a class-mate play the role of the patient and instruct him/her to follow only your instructions and not to anticipate what you will say. When you have finished, switch roles and recreate the situation.

B) Following Instructions

Number the phrases below from 1 to 10 to form a logical set of instructions. Then after you have finished, translate them from SPANISH to ENGLISH in the space provided below.

#	Instruction:	Translation:
____	*Permítame ponerle en la postura correcta.*	_____
____	*Desvístese y póngase esto, por favor.*	_____
____	*No respire.*	_____
____	*Soy el técnico.*	_____
____	*Voy a tomarle la radiografía ahora.*	_____
____	*Ahora, tome un respiro hondo.*	_____
____	*Gracias, hemos terminado.*	_____
____	*Póngase aquí con los brazos a los costados.*	_____
____	*Aguante la postura hasta que le diga que se relaje.*	_____
____	*Aguántelo.*	_____

Section III
The Blood Test

Phrases

English	Pronunciation & Spanish
1. I need to do a blood test on you.	*nay-say-**see**-toh ah-**sayr**-lay oon ah-**nah**-lee-sees day **sahn**-gray.* Necesito hacerle un análisis de sangre.
2. Have a seat.	***see^ayn**-tay-say pohr fah-**bohr**.* Siéntese, por favor.[1]
3. Relax.	*rray-**lah**-hay-say.* Relájese.
4. Roll up your sleeve.	***soo**-bah-say lah **mahn**-gah.* Súbase la manga.
5. Extend your arm and close your hand.	*ayk-**stee^ayn**-dah ayl **brah**-soh ee **see^ay**-rray lah **mah**-noh.* Extienda el brazo y cierre la mano.
6. Keep it closed and squeeze lightly.	*mahn-**tayn**-gah-lah say-**rrah**-dah ee ah-**pree^ay**-tay-lah lay-bay-**mayn**-tay.* Manténgala cerrada y apriétela levemente.
7. Don't move your arm, please.	*noh **mway**-bah ayl **brah**-soh pohr fah-**bohr**.* No mueva el brazo, por favor.
8. I'm going to put a tourniquet on you.	*lay boy ah poh-**nayr** oon tohr-nee-**kay**-tay.* Le voy a poner un torniquete.
9. I'm going to clean the area with a little alcohol.	*lay boy ah leem-**pee^ahr** ayl **see**-tee^oh kohn* Le voy a limpiar el sitio con *oon **poh**-koh day ahl-koh-**ohl**.* un poco de alcohol.
10. It may hurt a little.	*kee-sahs lay **bah**-yah ah doh-**layr** oon **poh**-koh.* Quizás le vaya a doler un poco.
11. Okay, open your hand.	*bee^ayn **ah**-brah lah **mah**-noh.* Bien, abra la mano.
12. Don't move your arm.	*noh **mway**-bah ayl **brah**-soh.* No mueva el brazo.
13. I'm going to take off the tourniquet.	*lay boy ah kee-**tahr** ayl tohr-nee-**kay**-tay.* Le voy a quitar el torniquete.
14. Bend your arm and press here with your fingers.	***doh**-blay ayl **brah**-soh ee ah-**pree^ay**-tay* Doble el brazo y apriete *ah-**kee** kohn lohs **day**-dohs.* aquí con los dedos.
15. I'm going to put a Band-Aid on it.	*lay boy ah poh-**nayr** **oo**-nah koo-**ree**-tah.* Le voy a poner una curita.[2]

16. Leave it on for a few minutes.	*day-hay-say lah koo-**ree**-tah doo-**rahn**-tay **bah**-ree^ohs mee-**noo**-tohs.* Déjese la curita durante varios minutos.[3]
17. I could not find the vein.	*noh **poo**-day ayn-kohn-**trahr** lah **bay**-nah.* No pude encontrar la vena.
18. I'm sorry, I need to do it again.	*loh **see**^**ayn**-toh loh nay-say-**see**-toh ah-**sayr** oh-**trah** bays.* Lo siento, lo necesito hacer otra vez.
19. We're done.	***ay**-mohs tayr-mee-**nah**-doh.* Hemos terminado.
20. Someone will call you with the results.	***ahl**-ghee^ayn lay yah-mah-**rah** kohn lohs rray-sool-**tah**-dohs.* Alguien le llamará con los resultados.

Notes

[1] Indicate where with a hand gesture.

[2] Use *algodón (ahl-goh-**dohn**)* instead of *una curita* if you are simply applying a cotton ball.

[3] Use *el algodón (ayl ahl-goh-**dohn**)* instead of *la curita* if you are using a cotton ball.

Practical Activities III

A) Oral Practice

Instructions: You are taking blood from a patient who speaks no ENGLISH and is rather nervous about the procedure. Relying on your knowledge from previous chapters, introduce yourself and say things to calm the patient. Then, explain the procedure as you perform it so the patient knows what to expect. Make sure your dialogue contains a minimum of 15 lines. Once you are prepared, form groups of four and have each pair recreate the situation for the other. If time permits, switch roles so that each person from each pair is patient and lab tech.

B) Following Instructions

Number the phrases below from 1 to 10 to form a logical set of instructions. Then after you have finished, translate them from SPANISH to ENGLISH in the space provided below.

#	Instruction:	Translation:
___	*Bien, abra la mano.*	_____
___	*Déjese el algodón durante varios minutos.*	_____
___	*Le voy a poner un torniquete.*	_____
___	*Súbase la manga.*	_____
___	*Manténgala cerrada y apriétela levemente.*	_____
___	*Extienda el brazo y cierre la mano.*	_____
___	*Quizás le vaya a doler un poco.*	_____
___	*Siéntese, por favor.*	_____
___	*Doble el brazo y apriete aquí con los dedos.*	_____
___	*Necesito hacerle un análisis de sangre.*	_____

Section IV
The Throat Culture

Phrases

English	Pronunciation & Spanish
1. The doctor has ordered a throat culture.	*ayl dohk-**tohr** ah pay-**dee**-doh oon kool-**tee**-boh day lah gahr-**gahn**-tah.* El doctor ha pedido un cultivo de la garganta.[1]
2. This will not hurt at all.	***ay**-stoh noh lay bah ah doh-**layr** pah-rah **nah**-dah.* Esto no le va a doler para nada.
3. Have a seat, please.	***see^ayn**-tay-say pohr fah-**bohr**.* Siéntese, por favor.[2]
4. I am going to use this to swab	*boy ah oo-**sahr** **ay**-stoh **pah**-rah froh-**tahr**-lay* Voy a usar esto para frotarle
your throat and tonsils.	*lah gahr-**gahn**-tah ee lahs ah-**meeg**-dah-lahs.* la garganta y las amígdalas.
5. Stick out your tongue and say "Ah."	***sah**-kay lah **layn**-gwah ee **dee**-gah ah.* Saque la lengua y diga "A".
6. Don't close your mouth.	*noh **see^ay**-rray lah **boh**-kah.* No cierre la boca.
7. It is common to want to gag.	*ays koh-**moon** kay-**rayr** ahr-kay-**ahr**.* Es común querer arquear.
8. That's it.	*ays **toh**-doh.* Es todo.
9. Someone will call you with the results.	***ahl**-ghee^ayn lay yah-mah-**rah** kohn lohs rray-sool-**tah**-dohs.* Alguien le llamará con los resultados.
10. In the mean time, gargle	***mee^ayn**-trahs **tahn**-toh **ah**-gah **gahr**-gah-ras* Mientras tanto, haga gárgaras
with warm salt water or	*kohn **ah**-gwah **tee**-bee^ah sah-**lah**-dah oh* con agua tibia salada o
use lozenges to alleviate	***choo**-pay pah-**stee**-yahs **pah**-rah swah-bee-**shar*** chupe pastillas para suavizar
any discomfort.	*ayl doh-**lohr** day gahr-**gahn**-tah.* el dolor de garganta.

Notes

[1] You may use *la doctora* instead of *el doctor* if you know the doctor to be female.

[2] Indicate where with a hand gesture.

Practical Activities IV

A) Oral Practice

Instructions: A patient has been sent to you for a throat culture. Prepare what you will say that explains the procedure as you perform it so the patient understands what is happening. Once you are prepared, form groups of four and have each pair recreate the situation for the other. If time permits, switch roles so that each person from each pair is patient and lab tech.

B) Matching

Instructions: Match the beginning of each phrase to the appropriate ending to form a complete sentence Afterwards, translate the phrases from SPANISH to ENGLISH. Do not worry about ordering the phrases for this exercise.

__ 1. Voy a usar esto . . .   a. gárgaras con agua tibia salada.

__ 2. Alguien le llamará . . .   b. todo.

__ 3. Mientras tanto, haga . . .   c. querer arquear.

__ 4. El doctor ha pedido . . .   d. con los resultados.

__ 5. Es . . .   e. la lengua y diga "A".

__ 6. Es común . . .   f. para fortarle la garganta y las amígdalas.

__ 7. Saque . . .   g. la boca.

__ 8. No cierre . . .   h. un cultivo de la garganta.

Translation:

1. _____

2. _____

3. _____

4. _____

5. _____

6. _____

7. _____

8. _____

9. _____

10. _____

Section V
The Stool Culture

Phrases

English	Pronunciation & Spanish
1. The doctor has ordered a stool culture.	*ayl dohk-**tohr** ah pay-**dee**-doh oon kool-**tee**-boh day ayk-skray-**mayn**-toh.* El doctor ha pedido un cultivo del excremento.[1]
2. Take this container (home) and	*yay-bay-say ay-stay frah-skoh (ah kah-sah) ee* Llévese este frasco (a casa) y
write your full name on it.	*ay-skree-bay soo nohm-bray kohm-play-toh ayn ayl.* escriba su nombre completo en él.[2]
3. Verify that this is your name.	*bay-ree-fee-kay kay ay-stay say^ah soo nohm-bray.* Verifique que éste sea su nombre.
4. The next time you have a bowel	*lah prohk-see-mah bays kay bah-yah day* La próxima vez que vaya de
movement, place a sample	*bee^ayn-tray pohn-gah oo-nah pay-kay-nyah* vientre, ponga una pequeña
(of your stool) in the container.	*mway-strah (dayl ayk-skray-mayn-toh) ayn ayl frah-skoh.* muestra (del excremento) en el frasco.[3]
5. Make sure the sample does not contain	*ah-say-goo-ray-say day kay noh ah-yah* Asegúrese de que no haya
toilet paper and that it	*pah-payl ee-hee-ay-nee-koh ayn lah mway-strah* papel higiénico en la muestra
has not been contaminated	*ee kay lah mway-strah noh ah-yah see-doh kohn-tah-mee-nah-dah* y que la muestra no haya sido contaminada
with urine.	*pohr oh-ree-nah.* por orina.
6. Place the container in this bag	*pohn-gah ayl frah-skoh ayn ay-stah bohl-sah ee* Ponga el frasco en esta bolsa y
and write your name on the bag.	*ay-skree-bah soo nohm-bray ayn lah bohl-sah.* escriba su nombre en la bolsa.
7. Then, bring us the sample	*loo^ay-goh trah^ee-gah-nohs lah mway-strah* Luego, tráiganos la muestra
(as soon as possible).	*(tahn prohn-toh koh-moh poh-see-blay).* (tan pronto como posible).
8. You may leave it at the front desk.	*pway-day day-hahr-lah ayn lah rray-sayp-see^ohn.* Puede dejarla en la recepción.
9. Someone will call you with the results.	*ahl-ghee^ayn lay yah-mah-rah kohn lohs rray-sool-tah-dohs.* Alguien le llamará con los resultados.

Notes

[1] You may use *la doctora* instead of *el doctor* if you know the doctor to be female.

[2] The following phrase is offered in the case that you are using a pre-printed label, in which case you would show the patient the printed information on the container.

[3] If . . . *vaya de vientre* . . . should still present a misunderstanding, the phrase . . . *vaya del dos* . . . *(bah-yah dayl dohs)* is also a commonly understood phrase but takes on a lower linguistic register, though it still avoids any potential vulgarity.

Practical Activities V

A) Oral Practice

Instructions: A patient has been sent to you for a stool culture. Prepare what you will say that gives the patient the necessary instructions for collecting and returning the sample. Once you are prepared, form groups of four and have each pair recreate the situation for the other. If time permits, switch roles so that each person from each pair is patient and lab tech.

B) Matching

Instructions: Match the beginning of each phrase to the appropriate ending to form a complete sentence. Afterwards, translate the phrases from SPANISH to ENGLISH. Do not worry about ordering the phrases for this exercise.

___ 1. Puede dejarla . . .

___ 2. Alguien le llamará . . .

___ 3. Asegúrese de que . . .

___ 4. El doctor ha pedido . . .

___ 5. Ponga el frasco . . .

___ 6. Verifique que . . .

___ 7. Luego, tráiganos . . .

___ 8. La próxima vez que vaya de vientre, . . .

a. no haya papel higiénico en la muestra.

b. un cultivo de excremento.

c. éste sea su nombre.

d. en la recepción.

e. la muestra tan pronto como posible.

f. ponga una pequeña muestra en el frasco.

g. con los resultados.

h. en esta bolsa y escríba su nombre en la bolsa.

Translation

1. _____

2. _____

3. _____

4. _____

5. _____

6. _____

7. _____

8. _____

9. _____

10. _____

...TON SCIENTIFIC HEALTH SCIENCES LIBRARY BROOKFIELD

Section VI
The Urine Test

Phrases

English	Pronunciation & Spanish
1. The doctor has requested a urinalysis.	*ayl dohk-**tohr** ah pay-**dee**-doh oon ah-**nah**-lee-sees day lah oh-**ree**-nah.* El doctor ha pedido un análisis de la orina.[1]
2. I am going to need a urine sample.	*boy ah nay-say-see-**tahr** **oo**-nah **mway**-strah day oh-**ree**-nah.* Voy a necesitar una muestra de orina.
3. Write your full name on this container.	*ay-**skree**-bay soo **nohm**-bray kohm-**play**-toh ayn **ay**-stay **frah**-skoh.* Escriba su nombre completo en este frasco.[2]
4. First, verify that this is your name.	*pree-may-roh bay-ree-**fee**-kay kay **ay**-stay say^ah soo **nohm**-bray.* Primero, verifique que éste sea su nombre.
5. Take the container to the restroom	***yay**-bay-say ayl **frah**-skoh ah lohs sayr-**bee**-see^ohs* Llévese el frasco a los servicios
and fill it (up to here) with urine.	*ee **yay**-nay-loh (**hoo**-stoh **ah**-stah ah-**kee**) kohn oh-**ree**-nah.* y llénelo (justo hasta aquí) con orina.[3]
6. Before urinating, thoroughly	***ahn**-tays day oh-ree-**nahr** leem-pee^ay-say bee^ayn* Antes de orinar, límpiese bien
clean your genitals with this.	*lohs hay-nee-**tah**-lays kohn **ay**-stoh.* los genitales con esto.[4]
7. Then, begin to urinate into the toilet.	*any-**tohn**-says koh-**mee^ayn**-say ah oh-ree-**nahr** ayn ayl ee-noh-**doh**-roh.* Entonces, comience a orinar en el inodoro.[5]
8. After a few seconds, urinate	*day-**spways** day **oo**-nohs say-**goon**-dohs tayr-**mee**-nay* Después de unos segundos, termine
in the container.	*day oh-ree-**nahr** ayn ayl **frah**-skoh.* de orinar en el frasco.[5]
9. Then, urinate into the container.	*ayn-**tohn**-says oh-**ree**-nay ayn ayl **frah**-skoh.* Entonces, orine en el frasco.
10. When you are finished, make sure the	***kwahn**-doh **ah**-yah tayr-mee-**nah**-doh **tah**-pay* Cuando haya terminado, tape
container is tightly closed.	*bee^ayn ayl **frah**-skoh.* bien el frasco.
11. Afterwards, leave it . . .	*day-**spways** loh bah ah day-**hahr** . . .* Después, lo va a dejar . . .
with me.	*kohn-**mee**-goh.* conmigo.
with the nurse on duty.	*kohn ayl ayn-fayr-**may**-roh day **gwahr**-dee^ah.* con el enfermero de guardia.

*kohn ayl **tayk**-nee-koh.*
with the lab tech.   con el técnico.

*ayn ayl lah-boh-rah-**toh**-ree^oh.*
in the lab.   en el laboratorio.

*ayn lah bayn-tah-**nee**-yah day lohs sayr-**bee**-see^ohs.*
on the counter in the restroom.   en la ventanilla de los servicios.

***ahl**-ghee^ayn lay yah-mah-**rah** kohn lohs rray-sool-**tah**-dohs.*
12. Someone will call you with the results.   Alguien le llamará con los resultados.

Notes

[1] You may use *la doctora* instead of *el doctor* if you know the doctor to be female.

[2] The following phrase is offered in the case that you are using a pre-printed label, in which case you would show the patient the printed information on the container.

[3] Point to the desired sample level on the container, if necessary.

[4] Hand the patient whatever items you want him/her to use.

[5] These two phrases have been included should you require a *midstream urine specimen*. Otherwise, you may skip them.

Practical Activities VI

A) Oral Practice

Instructions: You must explain to two different patients how to obtain a urine sample. The doctor has requested that PATIENT #1 collect a urine sample mid-stream while PATIENT #2 will not. Prepare what you will say to each patient, making the necessary changes to correctly communicate the doctor's specifications to each one. Once you are prepared, form groups of three. Using SPANISH only, give each patient the instructions for collecting the samples. After you have finished, ask the patients to tell you in ENGLISH, which one of them was PATIENT #1 (urine sample mid-stream). If time permits, switch roles so that each person has the chance to give and take instructions.

B) Matching

Match the beginning of each phrase to the appropriate ending to form a complete sentence. Afterwards, translate the phrases from SPANISH to ENGLISH. Do not worry about ordering the phrases for this exercise.

___ 1. Voy a necesitar . . .

___ 2. Antes de orinar, . . .

___ 3. Cuando haya terminado, . . .

___ 4. Después, lo va a dejar . . .

___ 5. Entonces, comience a . . .

___ 6. Entonces, orine . . .

___ 7. Llévese el frasco . . .

___ 8. Después de unos segundos, . . .

a. tape bien el frasco.

b. orinar en el inodoro.

c. en el frasco.

d. una muestra de orina.

e. con el enfermero de guardia.

f. termine de orinar en el frasco.

g. límpiese bien los genitales con esto.

h. a los servicios y llénelo con orina.

Translation:

1. _____

2. _____

3. _____

4. _____

5. _____

6. _____

7. _____

8. _____

Section VII
The Mammogram

Phrases

English	Pronunciation & Spanish
1. The doctor has requested a mammogram.	*ayl dohk-**tohr** ah pay-**dee**-doh oon mah-moh-**grah**-mah.* El doctor ha pedido un mamograma.[1]
2. You will need to make an appointment.	*nay-say-**see**-tah proh-grah-**mahr** oo-nah **see**-tah.* Necesita programar una cita.
3. Is this your first mammogram?	***ay**-stay ays soo pree-**mayr** mah-moh-**grah**-mah?* ¿Este es su primer mamograma?
4. When was your last mammogram?	*kwahn-**doh** lay ee-**see^ay**-rohn soo **ool**-tee-moh mah-moh-**grah**-mah?* ¿Cuándo le hicieron su último mamograma?
5. The day of your mammogram	*ayl **dee**-ah day soo mah-moh-**grah**-mah* El día de su mamograma,
don't use . . .	*noh **oo**-say . . .* no use . . .
any creams or lotions.	***kray**-mahs oh loh-**see^oh**-nays.* cremas o lociones.
deodorants.	*day-soh-doh-**rahn**-tays.* desodorantes.
body powder.	***tahl**-koh.* talco.
perfumes.	*payr-**foo**-mays.* perfumes.
6. The day of your mammogram	*ayl **dee**-ah day soo mah-moh-**grah**-mah* El día de su mamograma,
don't wear any jewelry.	*noh **yay**-bay **hoy**-yahs.* no lleve joyas.
7. Please remove any jewelry.	*fah-**bohr** day kee-**tahr**-say lahs **hoy**-yahs.* Favor de quitarse las joyas.
8. Undress to your waist, please.	*days-**noo**-day-say **ah**-stah lah seen-**too**-rah pohr fah-**bohr**.* Desnúdese hasta la cintura, por favor.
9. Please stand here facing the machine.	*fah-**bohr** day poh-**nayr**-say ah-**kee** ayn-**frayn**-tay day lah mah-**kee**-nah.* Favor de ponerse aquí enfrente de la máquina.
10. To do the mammogram,	***pah**-rah ah-**sayr**-lay ayl mah-moh-**grah**-mah* Para hacerle el mamograma,
I will need to flatten your breast	*boy ah nay-say-see-**tahr** ah-plah-**nahr**-lay ayl **say**-noh* voy a necesitar aplanarle el seno
as much as possible.	***tahn**-toh **koh**-moh poh-**see**-blay.* tanto como posible.

UNIVERSITY COLLEGE Library CORK

11. I am going to place your right/left breast

*boy ah poh-**nayr** ayl **say**-noh day-**ray**-choh / ees-**kee^ayr**-doh*
Voy a poner el seno derecho / izquierdo

between these two plates.

*ayn-tray **ay**-stahs dohs **plah**-kahs.*
entre estas dos placas.

12. Now, I am going to compress it.

*ah-**oh**-rah boy ah kohm-pree-**meer**-say-loh.*
Ahora, voy a comprimírselo.

13. You may be uncomfortable but

*pway-day kay ay-**stay** een-**koh**-moh-dah **pay**-roh*
Puede que esté incómoda pero

it is only temporary.

*ays **soh**-loh taym-poh-**rah**-nay^oh.*
es sólo temporáneo.

14. Don't move once I have positioned you.

*noh say **mway**-bah **oo**-nah bays kay lay **pohn**-gah ayn poh-**stoo**-rah.*
No se mueva una vez que le ponga en postura.

15. Raise your right/left arm and

*lay-**bahn**-tay ayl **brah**-soh day-**ray**-choh / ees-**kee^ayr**-doh*
Levante el brazo derecho/izquierdo

lean in toward the machine.

*ay een-**klee**-nay-say **ah**-see^ah lah **mah**-kee-nah.*
e inclínese hacia la máquina.

16. Hold the position and don't move.

*ah-**gwahn**-tay lah poh-**stoo**-rah ee noh say **mway**-bah.*
Aguante la postura y no se mueva.

17. Good. Now, I need to repeat the process

*bee^ayn. ah-**oh**-rah nay-say-**see**-toh rray-pay-**teer***
Bien. Ahora, necesito repetir el proceso

with the other breast.

*ayl proh-**say**-soh kohn ayl **oh**-troh say-noh.*
con el otro seno.

18. Please wait a moment,

*ay-**spay**-ray oon moh-**mayn**-toh pohr fah-**boh**r*
Espere un momento por favor,

I need to see if

*nay-say-**see**-toh sah-**bayr** kay lahs*
necesito saber que las

the x-rays turned out okay.

*rrah-dee^oh-grah-**fee**-ahs ahn sah-**lee**-doh bee^ayn.*
radiografías han salido bien.

19. I'm sorry, I need to take another x-ray

*loh **see^ayn**-toh nay-say-**see**-toh ah-**sayr**-lay **oh**-trah rrah-dee^oh-grah-**fee**-ah*
Lo siento, necesito hacerle otra radiografía

of the right/left breast.

*dayl **say**-noh day-**ray**-choh / ees-**kee^ayr**-doh.*
del seno derecho / izquierdo.

20. We're done.

*ay-mohs tayr-mee-**nah**-doh.*
Hemos terminado.

21. You may get dressed now.

*pway-day bay-**steer**-say ah-**oh**-rah.*
Puede vestirse ahora.

22. Someone will call you with the results.

*ahl-ghee^ayn lay yah-mah-**rah** kohn lohs rray-sool-**tah**-dohs.*
Alguien le llamará con los resultados.

Notes

[1] You may use *la doctora* instead of *el doctor* if you know the doctor to be female.

Practical Activities VII

A) Oral Practice

Instructions: A Hispanic patient has been scheduled for her first mammogram. Before meeting with the patient, there are several things you should consider regarding Hispanic females and procedures they may view as invassive. Talk this over with a few classmates and make a list of these items. Then, share your thoughts with the class. Finally, prepare a dialogue in which you greet the patient, make her feel more at ease and then give instructions for carrying out the procedure. Refer back to previous chapters if necessary for appropriate phrases and expressions.

B) Matching

Instructions: Match the beginning of each phrase to the appropriate ending to form a complete sentence. Afterwards, translate the phrases from SPANISH to ENGLISH. Then, write them below in ENGLISH in the most logical order.

___ 1. El día de su mamograma, . . .   a. y no se mueva.

___ 2. Favor de ponerse aquí . . .   b. vestirse ahora.

___ 3. Aguante la postura . . .   c. incómoda pero es sólo temporáneo.

___ 4. Voy a poner el seno . . .   d. programar una cita.

___ 5. Puede . . .   e. las joyas.

___ 6. No se mueva una vez . . .   f. la cintura, por favor.

___ 7. Desnúdese hasta . . .   g. enfrente de la máquina.

___ 8. Necesita . . .   h. derecho entre estas dos placas.

___ 9. Favor de quitarse . . .   i. no lleve joyas.

___ 10. Puede que esté . . .   j. que le ponga en postura.

Translation

1. _____

2. _____

3. _____

4. _____

5. _____

6. _____

7. _____

8. _____

9. _____

10. _____

Section VIII
Injections and IV

Phrases

English	Pronunciation & Spanish
1. I am going to give you an injection.	*lay boy ah dahr **oo**-nah een-yayk-**see^ohn**.* Le voy a dar una inyección.
2. I am going to start you on an IV.	*lay boy ah poh-**nayr** oon **sway**-roh.* Le voy a poner un suero.
3. It will help you with the pain.	*lay bah ah ah-lee-**bee^ahr** ayl doh-**lohr**.* Le va a aliviar el dolor.
4. The IV is not painful once it's in place.	***oo**-nah bays **pway**-stoh ayl **sway**-roh noh lay doh-lay-**rah**.* Una vez puesto, el suero no le dolerá.
5. Lie down.	*ah-**kway**-stay-say.* Acuéstese.
6. Lie still.	***kay**-day-say een-**moh**-beel.* Quédese inmóvil.
7. Roll up your sleeve.	***soo**-bah-say lah **mahn**-gah.* Súbese la manga.
8. Give me your arm.	***day**-may ayl **brah**-soh.* Déme el brazo.
9. You are going to feel a little stick.	*bah ah sayn-**teer** oon pay-**kay**-nyoh peen-**chah**-soh.* Va a sentir un pequeño pinchazo.
10. The IV is providing you with . . .	*ayl **sway**-roh ays **pah**-rah **dahr**-lay . . .* El suero es para darle . . .
food.	*day koh-**mayr**.* de comer.
medicine.	*may-dee-**see**-nah.* medicina.
11. This will help rehydrate you.	***ay**-stoh lay **bah** ah rray-ee-drah-**tahr**.* Esto le va a rehidratar.

Practical Activities VIII

A) Oral Practice

Instructions: Read each situation then prepare the instructions you will give the patient using only SPANISH. When you are ready, find a partner and have him/her play the role of patient while you play the role of health care professional. When you are done, switch roles and recreate each situation.

Patient #1 needs an injection to alleviate pain. Have the patient lie down and stay still. Explain that it may hurt a little. Afterwards, the patient will need an IV to continue the administration of the pain medicine. Tell the patient that once in place it doesn't hurt.

Patient #2 needs an IV for rehydration and to provide nutrients. Make sure the patient is lying down. Ask him/her to roll up a sleeve and give you the left arm. Also, the patient will need an injection to alleviate pain.

B) Matching

Instructions: Match the beginning of each phrase to the appropriate ending to form a complete sentence. Afterwards, translate the phrases from SPANISH to ENGLISH. Do not worry about ordering the phrases for this exercise.

___ 1. Déme . . .	a. inmóvil.
___ 2. Le voy a poner . . .	b. darle de comer.
___ 3. Le voy a dar . . .	c. rehidratar.
___ 4. Quédese . . .	d. el brazo.
___ 5. El suero es para . . .	e. la manga.
___ 6. Esto le va a . . .	f. aliviar el dolor.
___ 7. Súbese . . .	g. una inyección.
___ 8. Le va a . . .	h. un suero.

Translation

1. _____

2. _____

3. _____

4. _____

5. _____

6. _____

7. _____

8. _____

Section IX
Test Results

Phrases[1]

English	Pronunciation & Spanish
1. We have the results from your	*tay-**nay**-mohs lohs rray-sool-**tah**-dohs day soo(s)* Tenemos los resultados de su(s)
procedure(s).	*proh-say-dee-**mee^ayn**-toh(s).* procedimiento(s).
2. We need to repeat the procedure(s).	*nay-say-see-**tah**-mohs rray-pay-**teer**-lay ayl (lohs) proh-say-dee-**mee^ayn**-toh(s).* Necesitamos repetirle el (los) procedimiento(s).[2]
3. The results are	*lohs rray-sool-**tah**-dohs sah-**lee^ay**-rohn* Los resultados salieron
positive / negative / inconclusive.	*poh-see-**tee**-bohs / nay-gah-**tee**-bohs / een-kohn-kloo-**see**-bohs.* positivos / negativos / inconclusivos.
4. You will need to come into	*nay-say-see-tah-**rah** bay-**neer** ahl kohn-sool-**toh**-ree^oh* Necesitará venir al consultorio
the office to get the results	***pah**-rah rray-see-**beer** lohs rray-sool-**tah**-dohs* para recibir los resultados
of your procedure(s).	*dayl (day lohs) proh-say-dee-**mee^ayn**-toh(s).* del (de los) procedimiento(s).[3]
5. You will need to bring an interpreter	*nay-say-see-tah-**rah** trah-**ayr** ah **oon** een-**tayr**-pray-tay* Necesitará traer a un intérprete
with you to the appointment.	*ah lah **see**-tah.* a la cita.
6. You need to schedule a	*nay-say-see-tah-**rah** proh-grah-**mahr oo**-nah* Necesitará programar una
follow-up appointment	***see**-tah day say-ghee-**mee^ayn**-toh* cita de seguimiento
(as soon as possible).	*(day een-may-**dee^ah**-toh).* (de inmediato).
7. The results may be a false positive.	***pway**-day kay lohs rray-sool-**tah**-dohs say^ahn **oon** poh-see-**tee**-boh **fahl**-soh.* Puede que los resultados sean un positivo falso.
8. We are going to give you a referral.	***bah**-mohs ah **dahr**-lay **oo**-nah rray-koh-mayn-dah-**see^ohn**.* Vamos a darle una recomendación.
9. We are going to refer you to a dietician.	***bah**-mohs ah rray-fay-**reer**-lay ah oon dee^ay-**tees**-tah.* Vamos a referirle a un dietista.
10. We are going to send you to a specialist.	***bah**-mohs ah rray-fay-**reer**-lay ah oon ay-spay-see^ahl-**lee**-stah.* Vamos a referirle a un especialista.

11. We need to change your medication.	*nay-say-see-**tah**-mohs kahm-**bee^ahr**-lay lah may-day-**see**-nah.* Necesitamos cambiarle la medicina.
12. We need to increase/decrease	*nay-say-see-**tah**-mohs een-kray-mayn-**tahr** / dees-meen-**noo^eer*** Necesitamos incrementar / disminuir
the dosage.	*lah **doh**-sees.* la dosis.
13. You need some additional tests.	*nay-say-**see**-tahn ah-**sayr**-lay **oo**-nahs **proo^ay**-bahs ah-dee-see^oh-**nah**-lays.* Necesitan hacerle unas pruebas adicionales.
14. You must monitor your activity level	***day**-bay day kwee-**dahr** soo nee-**bayl** day ahk-tee-bee-**dahd*** Debe de cuidar su nivel de actividad
(carefully).	*(kohn kwee-**dah**-doh).* (con cuidado).
15. Call this number to set up	***yah**-may ah **ay**-stay **noo**-may-roh **pah**-rah proh-grah-**mahr*** Llame a este número para programar
your appointment.	*soo **see**-tah.* su cita.
16. We can call to set up the appointment	*poh-**day**-mohs yah-**mahr** pah-rah proh-grah-**mahr** lah **see**-tah* Podemos llamar para programar la cita
if you like.	*see kee-**see^ay**-rah.* si quisiera.

Notes

[1] The phrases and expressions in this chapter are intended to assist you in communicating in a general nature with the patient until a qualified interpreter can explain the detailed information.

[2] Use *el procedimiento* when singular. Use *los procedimientos* when plural.

[3] Use *del procedimiento* when singular. Use *de los procedimientos* when plural.

Practical Activities IX

A) Oral Practice

Instructions: Read each situation then prepare what you will tell the patient using only SPANISH. When you are ready, find a partner and present your dialogue as if (s)he were the patient. When you are done, switch roles and recreate each situation. Refer to previous chapters for any necessary phrases or expressions.

Patient #1

Call the patient and introduce yourself.
Tell the patient:

- you are calling on behalf of Dr. Smith.
- you are calling with the test results from _____ (choose a procedure from Chapter 10).
- the results are inconclusive.
- to make a follow-up appointment.
- the procedure will need to be repeated.
- to please bring an interpreter.

Patient #2

Call the patient and introduce yourself.
Tell the patient:

- you are calling with the results from _____ (choose a procedure from Chapter 10).
- the results are positive.
- to schedule follow-up appointment as soon as possible.
- to bring an interpreter.
- you are going to refer him/her to a specialist.
- to limit all physical activity.

B) Translation

Instructions: Read the dialogue below then translate it into ENGLISH in the space provided below.

"Buenos días. ¿Está la señora Gómez? . . . Buenos días señora Gómez. Soy —-. Llamo de parte del doctor Smith. Tenemos los resultados de su procedimiento. Los resultados para el cultivo de la garganta salieron positivos. Vamos a referirle a un especialista. Necesitará programar una cita de seguimiento de inmediato. Su número de teléfono es el 919-555-7586. La recepcionista habla español*. Gracias. Qué pase un buen día".

The receptionist speaks Spanish (lah rray-sayp-see^oh-nee**-stah **ah**-blah ay-spah-**nyol**).*

Chapter 11

Useful Commands for Many Commonly Encountered Situations

Phrases[1]

English	Pronunciation & Spanish
1. Stand (here/there).	*pohn-gah-say (ah-kee / ah-yee).* Póngase (aquí / allí).
2. Sit down.	*see^ayn-tay-say.* Siéntese.
3. Stand up.	*pohn-gah-say day pee^ay.* Póngase de pie.
4. Sit up.	*see^ayn-tay-say day-ray-choh/chah.* Siéntese derecho/a.
5. Lie face down.	*ah-kway-stay-say boh-kah ah-bah-hoh.* Acuéstese boca abajo.
6. Lie face up.	*ah-kway-stay-say boh-kah ah-rree-bah.* Acuéstese boca arriba.
7. Get up.	*lay-bahn-tay-say.* Levántese.
8. Relax.	*rray-lah-hay-say.* Relájese.
9. Breath deeply.	*rray-spee-ray ohn-doh.* Respire hondo.
10. Inhale.	*een-ah-lay.* Inhale.
11. Exhale.	*ayk-sah-lay.* Exhale.
12. Hold your breath.	*ah-gwahn-tay lah rray-spee-rah-see^ohn.* Aguante la respiración.
13. Roll over.	*day-say lah bwayl-tah.* Dése la vuelta.

14. Roll onto your right/left side.

*pohn-gah-say dayl koh-**stah**-doh day-**ray**-choh / ee-**skee**^ayr-doh.*
Póngase del costado derecho / izquierdo.

15. Bend over.

doh-blay-say.
Dóblese.

16. Stretch.

*ayk-**stee**-ray-say.*
Extírese.

17. Flex your (right/left) . . .

doh-blay . . .
Doble . . .

    arm.

*ayl **brah**-soh (day-**ray**-choh / ee-**skee**^ayr-doh).*
el brazo (derecho / izquierdo).

    leg.

*lah **pee**^ayr-nah (day-**ray**-chah / ee-**skee**^ayr-dah).*
la pierna (derecha / izquierda).

    knee.

*lah rroh-**dee**-yah (day-**ray**-chah / ee-**skee**^ayr-dah).*
la rodilla (derecha / izquierda).

    finger.

*ayl **day**-doh.*
el dedo.

18. Extend your (right/left) . . .

*ayk-**stee**^ayn-dah . . .*
Extienda . . .

    arm.

*ayl **brah**-soh (day-**ray**-choh / ee-**skee**^ayr-doh).*
el brazo (derecho / izquierdo).

    leg.

*lah **pee**^ayr-nah (day-**ray**-chah / ee-**skee**^ayr-dah).*
la pierna (derecha / izquierda).

    knee.

*lah rroh-**dee**-yah (day-**ray**-chah / ee-**skee**^ayr-dah).*
la rodilla (derecha / izquierda).

    finger.

*ayl **day**-doh.*
el dedo.

19. Raise your (right/left) . . .

*lay-**bahn**-tay . . .*
Levante . . .

    arm.

*ayl **brah**-soh (day-**ray**-choh / ee-**skee**^ayr-doh).*
el brazo (derecho / izquierdo).

    leg.

*lah **pee**^ayr-nah (day-**ray**-chah / ee-**skee**^ayr-dah).*
la pierna (derecha / izquierda).

    head.

*lah kah-**bay**-sah.*
la cabeza.

20. Close your (right/left) hand.

*see^**ay**-rray lah **mah**-noh (day-**ray**-chah / ee-**skee**^ayr-dah).*
Cierre la mano (derecha / izquierda).

21. Open your (right/left) hand.

*ah-brah lah **mah**-noh (day-**ray**-chah / ee-**skee**^ayr-dah).*
Abra la mano (derecha / izquierda).

22. Squeeze (as hard as you can).

*ah-**pree**^ay-tay (loh mahs kay **pway**-dah).*
Apriete (lo más que pueda).

23. Extend your fingers (one at a time).

*ayk-**stee^ayn**-dah lohs **day**-dohs (**oo**-noh ah lah bays).*
Extienda los dedos (uno a la vez).

24. Close your fingers (one at a time).

*see^**ay**-rray lohs **day**-dohs (**oo**-noh ah lah bays).*
Cierre los dedos (uno a la vez).

25. Release it.
[as in a grip with one's hand]

swayl-tay-loh.
Suéltelo.

26. Open your mouth.

*ah-brah lah **boh**-kah.*
Abra la boca.

27. Close your mouth.

*see^**ay**-rray lah **boh**-kah.*
Cierre la boca.

28. Look up / down / side to side.

*mee-ray ah-**rree**-bah / ah-**bah**-hoh / day oon **lah**-doh ah **oh**-troh.*
Mire arriba / abajo / de un lado a otro.

29. More.

mahs.
Más.

30. Less

may-nohs.
Menos.

31. Cough.

toh-sah.
Tosa.

32. Again.
[as in repeating an action]

oh-trah bays.
Otra vez.

33. Take this off.

*kee-tay-say **ay**-stoh.*
Quítese esto.

34. Put this on.

*pohn-gah-say **ay**-stoh.*
Póngase esto.

35. Turn around.

*day **oo**-nah **bwayl**-tah.*
Dé una vuelta.

36. Face me.

*pohn-gah-say ayn-**frayn**-tay day mee.*
Póngase enfrente de mí.

37. Walk.

*kah-**mee**-nay.*
Camine.

38. Be careful.

*tayn-gah kwee-**dah**-doh.*
Tenga cuidado.

39. Repeat. [as in information]

*rray-**pee**-tah.*
Repita.

40. Slowly.

*layn-tah-**mayn**-tay.*
Lentamente.

41. Quickly.

rrah-pee-dah-mayn-tay.
Rápidamente.

	*kohn kwee-**dah**-doh.*
42. Carefully.	Con cuidado.
	*proo-**dayn**-tay-**mayn**-tay.*
43. Cautiously.	Prudentemente.
	*. . . seen moh-**bayr** lah kah-**bay**-sah.*
44. . . . without moving your head.	. . . sin mover la cabeza.
	*ah-**see**.*
45. Like this.	Así.

Notes

[1] In addition to giving the command, you may want to act it out as well or use appropriate hand gestures to ensure deeper comprehension. Many of the commands are generic is structure and may require visual clarification. For example *Take this off* and *Put this on* would be better understood if the health care provider pointed to say, a shirt and then handed the patient a hospital gown. Also, as you learned earlier, the use of courtesy expressions, such as *por favor* and *gracias*, should be liberally interjected into conversations, especially when using commands.

Practical Activities

A) Oral Practice — Chain Effect

Instructions: For this activity, form groups of 3 to 5 people, depending upon the size of your class. Then, the instructor will divide the 45 commands from this chapter so that each group has approximately the same number but, of course, different commands. It is then the responsibility of each group and all of its members to thoroughly learn their assigned commands. To do this, have each group member be responsible for a phrase or set of phrases. That group member will then learn the phrases well enough to teach the other members of the group without relying on the text. Once each member has taught all of his/her phrases and the group itself has learned them relatively well, have each group then teach the other groups the phrases their members have learned. Thus, the chain effect begins with an inidividual learning a few phrases, teaching his/her other group members and finally, each group teaching the others. Since these are commands, it would be best to associate each command with the respective action, when possible, to facilitate retention.

B) Commands

Instructions: You may have noticed that the commands presented in this chapter are affirmative. However, you may need to use the negative form at some point. Following the examples below, write the negative forms of the affirmative commands given. To pronounce the negative command follow the pronunciation given for the affirmative form of the command you need and place *no (noh)* in the proper position. Your instuctor may also help you with this. Don't worry about accent marks since writing is not the primary focus. Look for a pattern in the following examples. Pay attention to what happens to the *se* when it is present. When you are finished, ask your instructor to review the correct responses.

	AFFIRMATIVE	NEGATIVE
1.	Siéntese.	No se siente.
2.	Acuéstese.	No se acueste.
3.	Póngase aquí.	No se ponga aquí.
4.	Levántese.	_____
5.	Extírese.	_____
6.	Dése la vuelta.	_____
7.	Relájese.	_____
8.	Quítese esto.	_____
9.	Respire hondo.	No respire hondo.
10.	Doble la rodilla.	No doble la rodilla.
11.	Abra la mano.	No abra la mano.
12.	Inhale.	_____
13.	Cierre los dedos.	_____
14.	Extienda el brazo.	_____
15.	Tosa.	_____
16.	Tenga cuidado.	_____

Chapter 12

Diagnosis and Common Medical Problems

Before You Begin

There are two very important cultural concepts that the health care professional should understand when diagnosing and/or treating a Hispanic patient, regardless of the patient's language abilities. These are *personalismo* *(payr-soh-nah-lees-moh)* and *familismo (fah-mee-lees-moh)*. In the Hispanic culture, *personalismo* is considered the "personal touch" that is expected from the health care professional. Although, this may seem to breach the barriers of formality of the Hispanic culture, it may be best understood as the "professional friendship" that exists between patient and health care professional. This expectation is carried over from the Hispanic culture's beliefs in *curanderismo* and *remedios caseros* (see *BEFORE YOU BEGIN from Chapter 9 - Assessing the Patient's Problem Preliminary Questions/Pain Assessment*). Alternately, *familismo* is described as the patient's entire family involved in the decision-making process regarding the patient's care and treatment. It is not uncommon that this may cause some delay in a patient's responsiveness to the health care provider's suggestions for treatment, etc., since the patient feels obligated to consult with family members before making any definitive decisions.

Many health care providers fail to realize that not only should oral communication reflect the values of *personalismo* and *familismo* but also that any media materials, such as translations or radio broadcasts should as well. This is especially critical in reaching the low-income, low-literacy portion of the underserved Hispanic population.

Phrases

English	Pronunciation & Spanish
1. We still don't know what is wrong.	*ah^oon noh sah-**bay**-mohs kwahl ays ayl proh-**blay**-mah.* Aún no sabemos cuál es el problema.
2. I believe we know what is wrong.	***kray**-oh kay sah-**bay**-mohs kwahl ays ayl proh-**blay**-mah.* Creo que sabemos cuál es el problema.
3. We are still trying to find the problem.	*ah^oon ay-**stah**-mohs trah-**tahn**-doh day ayn-tay-**rahr**-nohs dayl proh-**blay**-mah.* Aún estamos tratando de enterarnos del problema.
4. You are suffering from . . .	***ay-stah** soo-**free^ayn**-doh day . . .* Está sufriendo de . . .[1]
an abscess.	*oon ahb-**say**-soh.* un absceso.
anxiety.	*ahn-see^ay-**dahd.*** ansiedad.
asthma.	***ahs**-mah.* asma.

atrophy of the muscles.

*ah-troh-**fee**-ah day lohs **moo**-skoo-lohs.*
atrofía de los músculos.

bradycardia.

*brah-dee-**kahr**-dee^ah.*
bradicardia.

cardiac arrythmia.

*ah-**rreet**-mee^ah kahr-**dee**-ah-kah.*
arritmia cardíaca.

(chronic) fatigue.

*kahn-**sahn**-see^oh (**kroh**-nee-koh).*
cansancio (crónico).

a common cold.

*oon rrays-**free^ah**-doh.*
un resfriado.

conjunctivitis.

*kohn-hoon-tee-**bee**-tees.*
conjuntivitis.

dehydration.

*days-ee-drah-tah-**see^ohn**.*
deshidratación.

delirium.

*day-**lee**-ree^oh.*
delirio.

depression.

*day-pray-**see^ohn**.*
depresión.

dyspepsia.

*dees-**payp**-see^ah.*
dispepsia.

edema.

*ay-**day**-mah.*
edema.

frostbite.

*kay-mah-**doo**-rah day **free**-oh.*
quemadura de frío.

hardening of the skin.

*ayn-doo-ray-see-**mee^ayn**-toh day lah pee^ayl.*
endurecimiento de la piel.

irregular heart beat.

*lah-**tee**-doh ee-rray-goo-**lahr** dayl koh-rah-**sohn**.*
latido irregular del corazón.

heartburn.

*ahr-**dohr** ayn ayl ay-**stoh**-mah-goh.*
ardor en el estómago.

a (hiatal) hernia.

***oo**-nah **ayr**-nee^ah (ee-ah-**tahl**).*
una hernia (hiatal).

palpitation(s).

*pahl-pee-tah-**see^ohn**(-ays).*
palpitación(es).

hot flashes.

*foh-**gah**-hay.*
fogaje.[2]

indigestion.

*een-dee-hay-**stee^ohn**.*
indigestión.

inflammation.

*een-flah-mah-**see^ohn**.*
inflamación.

jaundice.

*eek-tay-**ree**-see^ah.*
ictericia.

locked jaw.

*mahn-**dee**-boo-lah say-**rrah**-dah.*
mandíbula cerrada.

locked knee.

*rroh-**dee**-yah bloh-kay-**ah**-dah.*
rodilla bloqueada.

menstruation problems.

*proh-**blay**-mahs day lah mayn-stroo^ah-**see**^ohn.*
problemas de la menstruación.

mental ability impairment.

*day-tay-**ree**^oh-roh day lah ah-bee-lee-**dahd** mayn-**tahl**.*
deterioro de la habilidad mental.

mononucleosis.

*moh-noh-noo-klay-**oh**-sees.*
mononucleosis.

paralysis.

*pah-**rah**-lee-sees.*
parálisis.

parasites.

*pah-**rah**-see-tohs.*
parásitos.

polyps.

***poh**-lee-pohs.*
pólipos.

pneumonia.

*pool-moh-**nee**-ah.*
pulmonía.

premature menopause.

*may-noh-**pah**^oo-see^ah pray-mah-**too**-rah.*
menopausia prematura.

premenstrual tension.

*tayn-**see**^ohn pray-mayn-**stroo**^ahl.*
tensión premenstrual.

prostration.

*proh-strah-**see**^ohn.*
prostración.

a pulmonary condition.

***oo**-nah kohn-dee-**see**^ohn pool-moh-**nahr**.*
una condición pulmonar.

rupture.

*rroop-**too**-rah.*
ruptura.

seizures.

*ah-**tah**-kays.*
ataques.

shock.

***choh**-kay.*
choque.

softening of the bones.

*rray-blahn-day-see-**mee**^ayn-toh day lohs **way**-sohs.*
reblandecimiento de los huesos.

softening of the nails.

*rray-blahn-day-see-**mee**^ayn-toh day lahs **oo**-nyahs.*
reblandecimiento de las uñas.

strep throat.

***oo**-nah een-fayk-**see**^ohn day gahr-**gahn**-tah pohr ay-strayp-toh-**koh**-kohs.*
una infección de garganta por estreptococos.

tachycardia.	*tah-kee-**kahr**-dee^ah.* taquicardia.
a tumor.	*oon too-**mohr**.* un tumor.
an ulcer.	***oo**-nah **ool**-say-rah.* una úlcera.
varicose veins.	***bay**-nahs bah-ree-**koh**-sahs.* venas varicosas.
a virus.	*oon **bee**-roos.* un virus.
warts.	*bay-**rroo**-gahs.* verrugas.
worms.	*lohm-**bree**-says.* lombrices.

Notes

[1] You may choose to give more detail by combining these phrases with specific body parts and organs found in Chapter 17. For example, to say *"You are suffering from a stomach ulcer."*, select the respective expression from this chapter and combine it with the appropriate phrase from Chapter 17 using the Spanish word *de*. You would then say *"Está sufriendo de una úlcera de estómago."* You may also use vocabulary presented in **Chapter 5 Medical History** for additional names of illnesses and diseases not listed here.

[2] An alternative expression for *hot flashes* is *bochorno (boh-**chohr**-noh)*.

Practical Activities

A) Oral Practice

Instructions: You have been reviewing lab results and chart notes for two patients. Now, you will need to contact each one and give him/her your diagnosis and any additional information necessary. Feel free to not only consult expressions from this chapter but from previous chapters as well. You may want to look ahead at Chapter 17 for additional terminology regarding body parts. After you have prepared your dialogue, present it to a classmate as if you were speaking to the patient.

Patient #1 (on the phone):

Greet the patient appropriately and identify yourself. Tell the patient:

- on whose behalf you are calling.
- you have the results of the blood work.
- the results are positive.
- the problem has been identified.
- you have (choose TWO health problems from #4 this chapter).
- to schedule a follow-up appointment.

Patient #2 (in the office):

Greet the patient and ask him/her to please follow you back to an exam room. Tell the patient:

- the results from the (choose a lab procedure from Chapter 10) were inconclusive.
- the problem still has not be identified.
- you are still trying to determine the problem.
- to schedule an appointment for some additional tests.

B) Putting It All Together

Instructions: In the oral exercise above, you were asked to combine phrases from this chapter with body parts from Chapter 17 in order to come up with more detailed information. Below, are several more ENGLISH combinations that you will need to figure out as well using the information from Chapter 17. For future reference, write them out in SPANISH. Then practice the pronunciation with a partner or as a class.

English: Spanish:

1. inflammation of the wrist _____

2. a mouth ulcer_____

3. a rupture of the spleen (ruptured spleen) _____

4. a hernia of the large intestine _____

5. an abcess of the brain (cerebral abcess) _____

6. parlysis in the legs_____

Cyber-Investigation

Launch an Internet search for Hispanics and Common Medical Problems. Then, search for statistical and factual information regarding Hispanics and their most common health-related issues. You may want to try expressing the search topic in a variety of ways, such as Hispanics and Health Problems, etc., to broaden your sources of information. Try to find, if possible, the top three medical problems of Hispanics. You may even choose to find additional information based on gender, age, etc. Share you findings with the class and compare it with the information found by others.

Chapter 13

Medication

Section I
Dosage Instructions

Before You Begin

It is very important to remember some general guidelines for numbers when writing them down for Hispanic patients. Remember that in Spanish, the decimal is used to write numbers whereas in English a comma is used. For example, the number 1.5 (or one and a half; one point five) in English would appear as 1,5 in Spanish. Likewise, larger numbers such as 2,550 (two thousand, five hundred fifty) as it appears in English, would be written as 2.550 in Spanish. However, do not let this overwhelm you as many Hispanics are quickly becoming accustomed to the English style of writing numbers.

Phrases

English	Pronunciation & Spanish
1. The doctor has prescribed medicine for you.	*ayl dohk-**tohr** / lah dohk-**toh**-rah lay ah rray-say-**tah**-doh may-dee-**see**-nah.* El doctor / la doctora le ha recetado medicina.
2. This is the prescription for the medicine.	***ay**-stah ays lah rray-**say**-tah **pah**-rah lah may-dee-**see**-nah.* Esta es la receta para la medicina.
3. These are the prescriptions for	***ay**-stahs sohn lahs rray-**say**-tahs **pah**-rah* Estas son las recetas para
your medicines.	*lahs may-dee-**see**-nahs.* las medicinas.
4. You can fill this (these) prescription(s)	***pway**-day soor-**teer ay**-stah(s) rray-**say**-tah(s)* Puede surtir esta(s) receta(s)
at any pharmacy.	*ayn kwahl-**kee^ayr** fahr-**mah**-see^ah.* en cualquier farmacia.
5. You need to fill this (these)	*nay-say-**see**-tah soor-**teer ay**-stah(s)* Necesita surtir esta(s)
prescription(s) at our pharmacy.	*rray-**say**-tah(s) ayn **noo^ay**-trah fahr-**mah**-see^ah.* receta(s) en nuestra farmacia.

6. This prescription is for . . .	*ay*-stah rray-**say**-tah ays **pah**-rah . . . Esta receta es para . . .[1]

7. These prescriptions are for . . .	*ay*-stahs rray-**say**-tahs sohn **pah**-rah . . . Estas recetas son para . . . [1]

8. It's a(n) . . .	*ays* . . . Es . . .
antibiotic.	ahn-tee-bee-**oh**-tee-koh. antibiótico.
antidiarrheal.	**pah**-rah ah-lee-**bee^ahr** lah dee^ah-**rray**-ah. para aliviar la diarrea.
antiemetic.	**pah**-rah ah-lee-**bee^ahr** lah **nah^oo**-see^ah ee ayl **boh**-mee-toh. para aliviar la náusea y el vómito.
anti-inflammatory.	**pah**-rah soo-pree-**meer** lah een-flah-mah-**see^ohn**. para suprimir la inflamación.
antitussive.	**pah**-rah rray-doo-**seer** lah tohs. para reducir la tos.
antiviral.	**pah**-rah kohm-bah-**teer** ayl **bee**-roohs. para combatir el virus.
bronchodilator.	**pah**-rah trah-**tahr** ayl **ahs**-mah. para tratar el asma.
decongestant.	days-koh-hays-tee^oh-**nahn**-tay. descongestionante.
diuretic.	**pah**-rah ah^oo-mayn-**tahr** lah proh-dook-**see^ohn** day oh-**ree**-nah. para aumentar la producción de orina.
emetic.	**pah**-rah proh-moh-**bayr** ayl **boh**-mee-toh. para promover el vómito.
expectorant.	ayk-spayk-toh-**rahn**-tay. expectorante.
hypnotic/soporific.	**pah**-rah een-doo-**seer** ayl **sway**-nyoh. para inducir el sueño.
laxative.	**pah**-rah trah-**tahr** ayl ay-stray-nyee-**mee^ayn**-toh. para tratar el estreñimiento.
painkiller.	**pah**-rah ah-lee-**bee^ahr** ayl doh-**lohr**. para aliviar el dolor.
stimulant.	ay-stee-moo-**lahn**-tay. estimulante.
tranquilizer.	trahn-kee-lee-**sahn**-tay. tranquilizante.

9. It comes in the form of . . .
*bee^**ay**-nay ayn **fohr**-mah day . . .*
Viene en forma de . . .

   pills.
*pah-**stee**-yahs.*
pastillas.[2]

   capsules.
kahp-soo-lahs.
cápsulas.

   syrup.
*hah-**rah**-bay.*
jarabe.

   an injection.
*een-yayk-**see^ohn**.*
inyección.

   a cream.
kray-mah.
crema.

   a powder.
pohl-boh.
polvo.

   an inhaler.
*een-ah-lah-**dohr**.*
inhalador.

   liquid.
lee-kee-doh.
líquido.

10. I'm going to explain the instructions.
*lay ayk-**splee**-koh lahs een-strook-**see^oh**-nays.*
Le explico las instrucciones.

11. Follow the instructions exactly.
*see-gah lahs een-strook-**see^oh**-nays ah-tayn-tah-**mayn**-tay.*
Siga las instrucciones atentamente.

12. Take . . . pill(s)/capsule(s)
*toh-may . . . pah-**stee**-yah(s) / **kahp**-soo-lah(s)*
Tome . . . pastilla(s) / cápsula(s)

   an eighth of a
*oon ohk-**tah**-boh day*
un octavo de

   a quarter of a
*oon **kwahr**-toh day*
un cuarto de

   half of a
may-dee^ah
media

   three quarters of a
*trays **kwahr**-tohs day*
tres cuartos de

   one
oo-nah
una

   two
dohs
dos

   three
trays
tres

	kwah-troh
four	cuatro

---

13. Take . . . teaspoon/tablespoon(s)	_toh_-may . . . koo-chah-rah-**dee**-tah(s) / koo-chah-**rah**-dah(s)
	Tome . . . cucharadita(s) / cucharada(s)
of the syrup / liquid	dayl hah-**rah**-bay / dayl **lee**-kee-doh (**kah**-dah)
	del jarabe / del líquido[4] (cada)
half of a	**may**-dee^ah
	media
one	**oo**-nah
	una
two	dohs
	dos
three	trays
	tres

---

14. Mix . . . teaspoon(s) / tablespoon(s)	**mays**-klay . . . koo-chah-rah-**dee**-tah(s) / koo-chah-**rah**-dah(s)
	Mezcle . . . cucharadita(s) / cucharada(s)
of the powder / liquid	dayl **pohl**-boh / dayl **lee**-kee-doh
	del polvo / del líquido
with water / milk / (orange) juice	kohn **ah**-gwah / **lay**-chay / **hoo**-goh (day nah-**rahn**-hah)
	con agua / leche / jugo (de naranja)
and take it	ee **toh**-may-loh (**kah**-dah)
	y tómelo[4] (cada)
one half	**may**-dee^ah
	media
one	**oo**-nah
	una
two	dohs
	dos
three	trays
	tres

---

15. Apply the cream/powder to	ah-**plee**-kay lah **kray**-mah / ayl **pohl**-boh **soh**-bray
	Aplique la crema / el polvo sobre
the affected area (every) . . .	ayl **ah**-ray-ah ah-fayk-**tah**-dah (**kah**-dah) . . .
	el área afectada (cada) . . . [4]

---

16. Use the inhaler (every) . . .	**oo**-say ayl een-ah-lah-**dohr** (**kah**-dah) . . .
	Use el inhalador (cada) . . . [4]

---

17. The injection is given (every) . . .	say ahd-mee-**nee**-strah lah een-yayk-**see**^ohn (**kah**-dah) . . .
	Se administra la inyección (cada) . . . [4]

18. (half) hour.

*(**may**-dee^ah) **oh**-rah.*
(media) hora.

    three hours.

*trays **oh**-rahs.*
tres horas.

    four hours.

***kwah**-troh **oh**-rahs.*
cuatro horas.

    once a day.

***oo**-nah bays ahl **dee**-ah.*
una vez al día.

    twice a day.

*dohs **bay**-says ahl **dee**-ah.*
dos veces al día.

    three times a day.

*trays **bay**-says ahl **dee**-ah.*
tres veces al día.

    four times a day.

***kwah**-troh **bay**-says ahl **dee**-ah.*
cuatro veces al día.

    in the morning.

*pohr lah mah-**nyah**-nah.*
por la mañana.

    in the afternoon.

*pohr lah **tahr**-day.*
por la tarde.

    in the evening.

*pohr lah **noh**-chay.*
por la noche.

    before a meal.

***ahn**-tays day koh-**mayr**.*
antes de comer.

    with a meal.

*kohn **oo**-nah koh-**mee**-dah.*
con una comida.

    after a meal.

*day-**spways** day koh-**mayr**.*
después de comer.

    with a glass of

*kohn (oon **bah**-soh day)*
con (un vaso de)

        water / milk / (orange) juice.

*ah-gwah / **lay**-chay / **hoo**-goh (day nah-**rahn**-hah).*
agua / leche / jugo (de naranja).

    on an empty stomach.

*kohn ayl ay-**stoh**-mah-goh bah-**see**-oh.*
con el estómago vacío.

    with a banana.

*kohn oon **plah**-tah-noh.*
con un plátano.[5]

    time you feel pain.

*bays kay **tayn**-gah doh-**lohr**.*
vez que tenga dolor.

    only if you are in pain.

***soh**-loh see **tee**^ay-nay doh-**lohr**.*
sólo si tiene dolor.

	*pohr ___ **dee**-ah(s).*
for ___ day(s).	por ___ día(s).[6]

	*pohr ___ **oh**-rah(s).*
for ___ hour(s).	por ___ hora(s).[6]

	*pway-day kohm-**prahr ay**-stah may-dee-**see**-nah*
19. You can buy this medicine	Puede comprar esta medicina

	*seen rray-**say**-tah **may**-dee-kah.*
without a prescription.	sin receta médica.

	*ah-say-**goo**-ray-say day toh-**mahr toh**-dah lah may-day-**see**-nah*
20. Make sure to take all of the medicine	Asegúrese de tomar toda la medicina

	*(**ah**-stah kay say lay ah-**kah**-bay).*
(until it is gone).	(hasta que se le acabe).

	*ah^oon-kay say **see**^ayn-tah may-**hohr**.*
even if you are feeling better.	aunque se sienta mejor.

	*see **pee**^ayr-day **oo**-nah **doh**-sees . . .*
21. If you miss a dose . . .	Si pierde una dosis . . .

	*noh **toh**-may **oo**-nah **ayk**-strah.*
don't take an extra dose.	no tome una extra.

	*toh-may-say-lah **kwahn**-toh **ahn**-tays.*
take it as soon as possible.	tómesela cuanto antes.

	*noh lah rray-koo-**pay**-ray.*
don't double up.	no la recupere.

	*see-gah kohn ayl oh-**rah**-ree^oh nohr-**mahl**.*
follow your normal schedule.	siga con el horario normal.

	yah-may-nohs.
call us.	llámenos.

Notes

[1] Use this phrase to introduce the name of the drug or drugs. For example, *"Esta receta es para bupropion".* Apply this to the plural phrase as well (when naming two or more drugs). For example, *"Estas recetas son para bupropion y fluoxetine".* Do not worry about the drug name in Spanish since the patient will need to become familiar with the English name.

[2] Another common word for *pastillas* is *píldoras (**peel**-doh-rahs).*

[3] Combine these expressions with the intervals of time given in #18 of this chapter. For example, to say *"Take half of a pill every three hours."* use *"Tome media pastilla cada tres horas"* and so on.

[4] Manipulate these phrases in the same manner by combining them with the intervals of time given in #18. For example, to say *"Take two tablespoons of the syrup in the morning for seven days."* use *"Tome dos cucharadas del jarabe por la mañana por siete días".* For more numbers, see Chapter 18.

[5] Another word for *plátano* is *banana (bah-**nah**-nah)* which of course is a more Americanized version.

[6] For numbers and pronunciation, see Chapter 18.

Practical Activities I

A) Oral Practice

Instructions: You are going to be giving various patients instructions on their medicines and dosage. Read the instructions provided in ENGLISH, then tell your patients in SPANISH what to do. Where indicated, choose the appropriate information to complete each set of instructions. However, do not recycle information. Each set of instructions MUST be different. Once you have prepared your instructions, present them to a small group and have them write them down in ENGLISH as they listen. Then, have them share what they wrote when you have finished to check their understanding.

PATIENT #1

Tell the patient:
- the doctor has precribed some medicine.
- this is the prescription for your medicine.
- which medicine the prescription is for.
- it can be filled at any pharmacy.
- the medicine's purpose (choose a medicine from #8 this chapter).
- the form of the medicine.
- how much to take, how often to take it and for how long.

PATIENTE #2

Tell the patient:
- the doctor has precribed some medicines.
- these are the precriptions for your medicines.
- what the two prescriptions are for.
- they need to be filled at the clinic's pharmacy.
- the purpose of the medicines (choose two medicines from #8 this chapter).
- the forms of the medicines.
- how much to take, how often to take it and for how long.
- what to do if a dose is missed.

PATIENT #3

Tell the patient:
- the doctor has precribed some medicines
- what the three prescriptions are for.
- one must be filled at the in-house pharmacy, another at any pharmacy and the last one is OTC.
- the purpose of the medicines (choose two medicines from #8 this chapter).
- the forms of the medicines (one liquid, one pill and one powder).
- how much to take, how often to take it and for how long.

B) Dosage Instructions

Instructions: Translate the SPANISH dosage instructions into ENGLISH either orally or in writing. Share your translation with a partner when you have finished. Help each other make any necessary adjustments before consulting the text.

Estas recetas son para Azithromycin y Dolasetron. Azithromycin es antibiótico y Dolasetron es para aliviar la náusea y el vómito. Azithromycin viene en forma de cápsulas y Dolasetron viene en forma de líquido. Tome dos cápsulas dos veces al día por diez días. Tome las cápsulas con una comida. Mezcle una cucharada del líquido con jugo de naranja y tómelo por la mañana con el estómago vacío. Asegúrese de tomar toda la medicina hasta que se le acabe aunque se sienta mejor. Si pierde una dosis no la recupere, siga con el horario normal.

Section II
Possible Side Effects

Phrases

English	Pronunciation & Spanish
1. The medicine may have side effects.	*lah may-day-**see**-nah **pway**-day tay-**nayr** ay-**fayk**-tohs say-koon-**dah**-ree^ohs.* La medicina puede tener efectos secundarios.
2. You may experience . . .	***pway**-day ayk-spay-ree-mayn-**tahr** . . .* Puede experimentar . . .
dry mouth.	*lah **boh**-kah **say**-kah.* la boca seca.
nausea (and vomiting).	***nah^oo**-see^ah (ee **boh**-mee-toh).* náusea (y vómito).
depression.	*lah day-pray-**see^ohn**.* la depresión.
irritability.	*lah ee-rree-tah-bee-lee-**dahd**.* la irritabilidad.
blurred/double vision.	*lah **bee**-stah boh-**rroh**-sah / **doh**-blay.* la vista borrosa / doble.
lack of appetite.	*lah **fahl**-tah day ah-pay-**tee**-toh.* la falta de apetito.
sleeplessness.	*ayl een-**sohm**-nee^oh.* el insomnio.
drowsiness.	*lah sohm-noh-**layn**-see^ah.* la somnolencia.
hair loss.	*lah **payr**-dee-dah day **pay**-loh.* la pérdida de pelo.
hunger/thirst.	*ayl **ahm**-bray / lah sayd.* el hambre / la sed.
constipation.	*ayl ay-stray-nyee-**mee^ayn**-toh.* el estreñimiento.
diarrhea.	*lah dee^ah-**rray**-ah.* la diarrea.
a bad taste in your mouth.	*oon mahl sah-**bohr** ayn lah **boh**-kah.* un mal sabor en la boca.
fatigue.	*lah fah-**tee**-gah.* la fatiga.
memory problems.	*proh-**blay**-mahs day may-**moh**-ree^ah.* problemas de memoria.

dizziness.	*ayl mah-**ray**-oh.* el mareo.
fainting.	*ayl days-**mah^ee**-yoh.* el desmayo.
ringing in the ears.	*ayl soom-**bee**-doh ayn lohs oh-**ee**-dohs.* el zumbido en los oídos.
indigestion.	*lah een-dee-hay-**stee^ohn**.* la indigestión.
frequent urination.	*ayl oh-ree-**nahr** kohn fray-**kwayn**-see^ah.* el orinar con frecuencia.
weakness.	*lah day-bee-lee-**dahd**.* la debilidad.
redness of the skin.	*ayl rroo-**bohr**.* el rubor.
swelling.	*ayl een-chah-**sohn**.* el hinchazón.
euphoria.	*lah ay^oo-**foh**-ree^ah.* la euforia.
high/low blood pressure.	*lah pray-**see^ohn ahl**-tah / **bah**-hah.* la presión alta / baja.
rash.	*oon sahl-poo-**yee**-doh.* un salpullido.
chills.	*ay-skah-loh-**free**-ohs.* escalofríos.

3. It may cause a(n) . . . infection.	***pway**-day kay **kah^oo**-say **oo**-nah een-fayk-**see^ohn** . . .* Puede que cause una infección . . .
viral	***bee**-rahl.* viral.
pulmonary	*pool-moh-**nahr**.* pulmonar.
respiratory	*rray-spee-rah-**toh**-ree^ah.* respiratoria.
kidney	*rray-**nahl**.* renal.
sinus	*see-noo-**sahl**.* sinusal.

4. If you experience a bad reaction	*see **tee^ay**-nay **oo**-nah rray-ahk-**see^ohn** ahd-**bayr**-sah* Si tiene una reacción adversa
to the medicine . . .	*ah lah may-dee-**see**-nah . . .* a la medicina . . .

call us.	*yah*-may-nohs. llámenos.
come back.	*rray*-**gray**-say. regrese.
go to the hospital (immediately).	*bah*-yah ahl oh-spee-**tahl** (day een-may-**dee^ah**-toh). vaya al hospital (de inmediato).
stop taking it.	*day*-hay day toh-**mahr**-lah. deje de tomarla.

5. Keep the medication out of the

mahn-**tayn**-gah lah may-dee-**see**-nah **fway**-rah dayl
Mantenga la medicina fuera del

reach of children (and pets).

ahl-**kahn**-say day lohs **nee**-nyohs (ee lahs mah-**skoh**-tahs).
alcance de los niños (y las mascotas).

6. If you have any questions

see **tee^ay**-nay ahl-**goo**-nahs pray-**goon**-tahs
Si tiene algunas preguntas

(or concerns), call us.

*(oh een-kee^ay-**too**-days)* **yah**-may-nohs.
(o inquietudes), llámenos.

Practical Activities II

A) Oral Practice

Instructions: You have just given some patient instructions on medication dosage. Now, you want to be sure to warn them of the possible side effects and what they should do if they experience them. Following the information below for each patient, prepare what you will say using only SPANISH. Complete information for the first two patients has been provided for you. You will need to fill in the missing information for the the third one. You may consult the last section and/or previous chapters for additional phrases. When you are ready, form a group of four and present each dialogue to a different group member as if (s)he were the patient. The group members should make notes in ENGLISH to check their comprehension. After you have finished, have them tell you what you understood.

PATIENT #1
Tell the patient:
- the medication has possible side effects.
- (s)he may experience dry mouth, lack of appetite, thirst, memory problems and frequent urination.
- if you experience a bad reaction to the medicine, stop taking it and go to the hospital.

PATIENTE #2
Tell the patient:
- the doctor has prescribed you some medicines.
- one prescription is for valsarten which is a highblood pressure medication.
- it has possible side effects.
- it may cause fatigue or abdominal pain.
- the other prescription is for ezetimibe/simvastatin and is for high cholesterol.
- it may cause headache or respiratory infection.

PATIENT #3
Tell the patient:
- the medication is for —
- it has possible side effects.
- you may experience _____ and _____.
- it may cause _____.
- if you experience a bad reaction, _____.*
  *Prepare this based on a real drug or one you "invent."

B) Warning of Potential Side Effects

Instructions: Translate the SPANISH information regarding this medication's side effects into ENGLISH either orally or in writing. Share your translation with a partner when you have finished. Help each other make any necessary adjustments before consulting the text.

La medicina puede tener efectos secundarios. Puede experimentar la irritabilidad, el insomnio, el estreñimiento y escalofríos. También (also), puede que cause una infección viral o respiratoria. Si tiene una reacción adversa a la medicina, vaya al hospital de inmediato. Mantenga la medicina fuera del alcance de los niños y las moscotas. Si tiene algunas preguntas o inquietudes, llámenos.

Chapter 14

Wound Care, Fractures, and Sprains

Phrases

English	Pronunciation & Spanish
1. You are going to need . . .	*bah ah nay-say-see-**tahr*** . . . Va a necesitar . . .
a bandage.	***oo**-nah **bayn**-dah.* una venda.[1]
a cast.	*oon **yay**-soh.* un yeso.[2]
a sling.	*oon kah-bay-**stree**-yoh.* un cabestrillo.
a splint.	***oo**-nah tah-**blee**-yah.* una tablilla.
stitches.	***poon**-tohs.* puntos.[3]
2. I am going to apply a(n) . . .	*lay boy ah ah-plee-**kahr oo**-nah* Le voy a aplicar una
compress.	*kohm-**pray**-sah* . . . compresa . . .
heat.	*kah-**lee^ayn**-tay.* caliente.
cold.	***free**-ah.* fría.
ice.	*day **ee^ay**-loh.* de hielo.
3. I need to clean the wound.	*nay-say-**see**-toh leem-**pee^ahr**-lay lah ay-**ree**-dah.* Necesito limpiarle la herida.
4. I'm going to have to move you.	***tayn**-goh kay moh-**bayr**-lay.* Tengo que moverle.
5. This may be (somewhat) uncomfortable.	***pway**-day kay **ays**-toh **say**-ah (oon **poh**-koh) een-**koh**-moh-doh.* Puede que esto sea (un poco) incómodo.
6. It appears you have. . . .	*pah-**ray**-say kay **tee^ay**-nay* . . . Parece que tiene . . .

a fracture.	*oo-nah frahk-**too**-rah.* una fractura.
a sprain.	*oo-nah tohr-say-**doo**-rah.* una torcedura.
a break.	*oo-nah kay-brah-**doo**-rah.* una quebradura.
a pulled muscle.	*oon **moo**-skoo-loh rahs-**gah**-doh.* un músculo rasgado.
a torn ligament.	*oon lee-gah-**mayn**-toh **rroh**-toh.* un ligamento roto.
a dislocated joint.	*oo-nah dees-loh-kah-**see^ohn**.* una dislocación.[4]
a puncture wound.	*oo-nah ay-**ree**-dah payr-foh-**rah**-dah.* una herida perforada.
a (serious) burn.	*oo-nah kay-mah-**doo**-rah (**say**-ree^ah).* una quemadura (seria).[5]
an animal bite.	*oo-nah mohr-**dee**-dah.* una mordida.
an insect bite.	*oo-nah pee-kah-**doo**-rah.* una picadura.
abrasions.	*ah-brah-**see^oh**-nays.* abrasiones.
lacerations.	*lah-say-rah-**see^oh**-nays.* laceraciones.

7. You will have to change the dressing periodically.	*tayn-**drah** kay kahm-**bee^ahr**-say lahs **bayn**-dahs* Tendrá que cambiarse las vendas *day **kwahn**-doh ayn **kwahn**-doh.* de cuando en cuando.
8. Watch what I do so you will know what to do at home.	*ohb-**sayr**-bay loh kay **ah**-goh **pah**-rah* Observe lo que hago para *kay **say**-pah kay ah-**sayr** ayn **kah**-sah.* que sepa qué hacer en casa.
9. Change the dressing . . .	*kahm-**bee^ay**-say lahs **bayn**-dahs . . .* Cámbiese las vendas . . . [6]
10. If the dressing is too tight, loosen it a little.	*see lahs **bayn**-dahs lay **kay**-dahn day-mah-**see^ah**-doh ah-pray-**tah**-dahs,* Si las vendas le quedan demasiado apretadas, *swayl-tay-lahs oon **poh**-koh.* suéltelas un poco.
11. Use compresses . . .	*oo-say kohm-**pray**-sahs . . .* Use compresas . . . [6]

12. Soak the affected area . . .

*rray-**moh**-hay lah **pahr**-tay ah-fayk-**tah**-dah . . .*
Remoje la parte afectada . . .

   in warm water.

*ayn **ah**-gwah **tee**-bee^ah.*
en agua tibia.

   in cold water.

*ayn **ah**-gwah **free**-ah.*
en agua fría.

13. You will need to elevate . . .

*nay-say-see-tah-**rah** ay-lay-**bahr** . . .*
Necesitará elevar . . .[6]

   your foot.

ayl pee^ay.
el pie.

   your arm.

*ayl **brah**-soh.*
el brazo.

   your hand.

*lah **mah**-noh.*
la mano.

   your head.

*lah kah-**bay**-sah.*
la cabeza.

14. Don't let the . . . get wet.

*noh **day**-hay kay say **moh**-hay . . .*
No deje que se moje . . .

   the cast

*ayl **yay**-soh.*
el yeso.

   the bandage

*lah **bayn**-dah.*
la venda.

15. Call us if the affected area . . .

*yah-may-nohs see ayl **ah**-ray-ah ah-fayk-**tah**-dah . . .*
Llámenos si el área afectada . . .

   changes color.

*kahm-bee^ay day koh-**lohr**.*
cambia de color.

   starts to drain.

*aym-**pee^ay**-sah ah dray-**nahr**.*
empieza a drenar.

   starts to bleed.

*aym-**pee^ay**-sah ah sahn-**grahr**.*
empieza a sangrar.

   swells.

*say **een**-chah.*
se hincha.

   becomes numb.

*say ayn-too-**may**-say.*
se entumece.

   becomes more painful.

*say **poh**-nay mahs doh-loh-**roh**-sah.*
se pone más dolorosa.

Notes

[1] An alternate word for *bandage* is *vendaje (bayn-**dah**-hay)* and would take *un (oon)* instead of *una (**oo**-nah)* here.

[2] An alternate word for *cast* is *escayola (ays-kah^ee-yoh-lah)* and would take *una (oo-nah)* instead of *un (oon)* here.

[3] An alternate word for *puntos* is *suturas (soo-too-rahs)*.

[4] An alternate word for *dislocation* is *luxación (look-sah-see^ohn)* and would take *una (oo-nah)* instead of *un (oon)* here.

[5] To indicate the degree of the burn use *quemadura* then add *de primer grado (day pree-mayr grah-doh), de segundo grado (day say-goon-doh grah-doh)* or *de tercer grado (day tayr-sayr grah-doh).* For example, *una quemadura de primer grado.*

[6] Use the instructions for *medication dosage* from Chapter 13 to detail how often if necessary.

Practical Activities

A) Oral Practice

Instructions: You are working in an urgent care clinic when someone rushes in with an injury requiring immediate attention. From the list, choose an injury and prepare what you would say to that individual in no less than 10 lines of dialogue. You may use expresssions and phrases from previous chapters is you wish (such as giving someone something for pain, etc.). Once you are prepared, find a partner and have that person play the injured patient (who does not need to speak). Recreate the scene for another pair once you have practiced. When finished, switch roles and allow your partner to present his/her dialogue. Onlookers should take notes as to what they believe is happening and share this with each pair after they present to verify their information.

Choose one of the following injuries upon which to base your dialogue:

- broken leg
- dislocated shoulder
- deep puncture wound
- torn ligament

- fractured ribs
- third degree burn
- severe skin lacerations
- sprained wrist

B) Matching

Instructions: Match the ENGLISH word from column B with the SPANISH word from column A. Check your answers when you have finished by looking back in the chapter at their meanings.

	A		B
____	1. cabestrillo	a.	insect bite
____	2. quemadura	b.	cast
____	3. mordida	c.	warm
____	4. tablilla	d.	dislocation
____	5. herida	e.	dressings
____	6. escayola	f.	painful
____	7. vendaje	g.	sling
____	8. vendas	h.	splint
____	9. compresa	i.	cold
____	10. picadura	j.	ice
____	11. hielo	k.	animal bite
____	12. luxación	l.	wound
____	13. dolorosa	m.	compress
____	14. tibia	n.	bandage
____	15. fría	o.	burn

Chapter 15

Standard Medical Forms

Section I
Medical Consent Form

Before You Begin

Many Hispanic immigrants speak little or no English and may even have a low literacy level in their native language. This, of course, can greatly impact the medical care they receive. It has been determined that among the continually increasing Hispanic population, the literacy level is comensarate with an individual's health. Those who primarily speak Spanish are at a greater risk for health problems than those who have some knowledge of English due to the language barrier. However, a direct correlation between a rise in the quality of medical care provided was noted when language services in Spanish were made available.

A Hispanic who is not very literate in Spanish, may print his/her name or use a symbol or set of symbols as his/her signature. Likewise, those who are completely literate may sign with a highly stylized signature which may not resemble their name at all.

Phrases

English	Pronunciation & Spanish
1. This is the medical consent	*ay-stay ays ayl fohr-moh-lah-ree^oh day kohn-sayn-tee-mee^ayn-toh pah-rah* Este es el formulario de consentimiento para
form. Please read it. Then	*trah-tah-mee^ayn-toh may-dee-koh. fah-bohr day lay-ayr-loh. loo^ay-goh* tratamiento médico. Favor de leerlo. Luego,
sign and date it.	*feer-may-loh ee fay-chay-loh.* fírmelo y féchelo.
2. Bring it to me when you have finished.	*trah^ee-gah-may-loh kwahn-doh ah^ee-yah tayr-mee-nah-doh.* Tráigamelo cuando haya terminado.
3. I can read it to you if you like.	*say loh pway-doh lay-ayr see kee^ay-ray.* Se lo puedo leer si quiere.
4. Please sign here, indicating	*fah-bohr day feer-mahr ah-kee een-dee-kahn-doh* Favor de firmar aquí,indicando
your consent to medical treatment.	*ayl kohn-sayn-tee-mee^ayn-toh pah-rah trah-tah-mee^ayn-toh may-dee-koh.* el consentimiento para tratamiento médico.

5. Do you understand that by signing

*kohm-**prayn**-day kay ahl feer-**mahr***
¿Comprende que al firmar

this form you give permission

***ay**-stay fohr-moo-**lah**-ree^oh dah payr-**mee**-soh*
este formulario, da permiso

to receive medical treatment?

***pah**-rah rray-see-**beer** trah-tah-**mee^ayn**-toh **may**-dee-koh?*
para recibir tratamiento médico?

6. (Pronunciation guide for Spanish Medical Consent Form)

CONSENTIMIENTO PARA TRATAMIENTO MEDICO

*yoh (1) [patient name] pohr lah pray-**sayn**-tay soh-lee-**see**-toh ee doy kohn-sayn-tee-**mee^ayn**-toh **pah**-rah kay lohs proh-fay-see^oh-**nah**-lays*
Yo (1) _____ por la presente solicito y doy consentimiento para que los profesionales

may**-dee-kohs day (2) [business name] ee soos ah-fee-**lee^ah**-dohs nohs ahd-mee-**nee**-strayn ah mee fah-**mee**-lee^ah ee ah mee kwahl-**kee^ayr
médicos de (2) _____ y sus afiliados nos administren a mi familia y a mí cualquier

*trah-tah-**mee^ayn**-toh **may**-dee-koh kohn-see-day-**rah**-doh nay-say-**sah**-ree^oh say-**goon** ayl may-**hohr** whee-**see^oh** day **dee**-chos*
tratamiento médico considerado necesario según el mejor juicio de dichos

*proh-fay-see^oh-**nah**-lays.*
profesionales.

***nohm**-bray (fah-**bohr** day ay-skree-**beer** ayn **lay**-trahs day **mohl**-day)*
nombre (favor de escribir en letras de molde): _____

***feer**-mah:*   *pah-rayn-**tay**-skoh ahl pah-**see^ayn**-tay:*
firma: _____ parentesco al paciente: _____

***fay**-chah:*
fecha: _____

Notes

The pronunciation guide need not be learned like the expressions presented in the other chapters. It is only provided to aid the health care provider in assisting illiterate patients or patients that may be visually impaired.

(Spanish version)

CONSENTIMIENTO PARA TRATAMIENTO MEDICO

Yo (1) _____ por la presente solicito y doy consentimiento para que los profesionales médicos de (2) _____ y sus afiliados nos administren a mi familia y a mí cualquier tratamiento médico considerado necesario según el mejor juicio de dichos profesionales.

nombre (favor de escribir en letras de molde): _____

firma: _____ parentesco al paciente: _____

fecha: _____

(English version)

CONSENT TO MEDICAL TREATMENT

I (1) _____ hereby request and give authorization to the medical professionals of (2) _____ and its affiliates to administer to my family and myself any medical treatment considered necessary according to the best judgement of said professionals.

name (please print):_____

signature: _____relation to patient: _____

date: _____

Using this form: The (1) requires that the consenting adult write his/her name, whereas (2) requires the name of the medical facility providing treatment.

* This page is an example provided for instructional purposes.

Practical Activities I

A) Oral Practice

Instructions: With a partner, practice reading the pronunciation guide for the Spanish Medical Consent Form aloud. Try doing this together first, then take turns reading it aloud to one another seperately. Remember, it does not have to be memorized. Afterwards, prepare the two situations given below individually, then present them to one another. Consult past chapters if necessary.

B) Translation

Instructions: Translate the following dialogue between a patient (P) and health care provider (HP). When you have finished, find a partner and compare your translations.

P - Buenos días. _____

HP - Hola. ¿En qué puedo servirle, señor? _____

P - Quiero ver a un doctor, por favor. _____

HP - ¿Esta es su primera cita con nosotros? _____

P - Sí, señorita. _____

HP - ¿Habla inglés? _____

P - Un poco. _____

HP - ¿Sabe leer y escribir? _____

P - No. _____

HP - Este es el fomulario de consentimiento para tratamiento médico. Se lo puede leer si quiere. _____

_____

P - Sí, por favor. _____

HP - (*Reads the consent form aloud.*) ¿Comprende que al firmar este formulario, da permiso para recibir

tratamiento médico? _____

P - Sí, comprendo. _____

HP - Muy bien. Puede esperar en la sala de espera. Le llaman en un momento. _____

_____

P - Bien. Gracias. _____

HP - De nada. _____

Section II
Medical Information Consent Release Form

Phrases

English	Pronunciation & Spanish
1. This is the consent to release of medical	*ay*-stay ays ayl fohr-moh-*lah*-ree^oh day Este es el formulario de
information form.	kohn-sayn-tee-*mee^ayn*-toh *pah*-rah lah dee-bool-gah-*see^ohn* consentimiento para la divulgación
Please read it.	day een-fohr-mah-*see^ohn may*-dee-kah. fah-*bohr* day lay-*ayr*-loh. de información médica. Favor de leerlo.
Then sign and date it.	*loo^ay*-goh *feer*-may-loh ee *fay*-chay-loh. Luego, fírmelo y féchelo.
2. Bring it to me when you have finished.	*trah^ee*-gah-may-loh *kwahn*-doh *ah^ee*-yah tayr-mee-*nah*-doh. Tráigamelo cuando haya terminado.
3. I can read it to you if you like.	say loh *pway*-doh lay-*ayr* see *kee^ay*-ray. Se lo puedo leer si quiere.
4. Please sign here, indicating	fah-*bohr* day feer-*mahr* ah-*kee* een-dee-*kahn*-doh Favor de firmar aquí, indicando
your consent to the release	ayl kohn-sayn-tee-*mee^ayn*-toh *pah*-rah lah dee-bool-gah-*see^ohn* el consentimiento para la divulgación
of medical information.	day een-fohr-mah-*see^ohn may*-dee-kah. de información médica.
5. Do you understand that by	kohm-*prayn*-day kay ahl feer-*mahr* ¿Comprende que al firmar
signing this you give us	*ay*-stay fohr-moo-*lah*-ree^oh nohs dah payr-*mee*-soh este formulario, nos da permiso
permission to release your	*pah*-rah kohm-pahr-*teer* lah een-fohr-mah-*see^ohn* para compartir la información
medical information according	*may*-dee-kah say-*goon* lohs *tayr*-mee-nohs médica según los términos
to the terms of the form?	een-dee-*kah*-dohs ayn ayl fohr-moo-*lah*-ree^oh? indicados en el formulario?

6. (Pronunciation guide for Spanish Medical Information Consent Release Form)

---

kohn-sayn-tee-mee^ayn-toh pah-rah lah dee-bool-gah-see^ohn day een-fohr-mah-see^ohn may-dee-kah
CONSENTIMIENTO PARA LA DIVULGACION DE INFORMACION MEDICA

(proh-tay-hee-dah pohr lah lay^ee)
(PROTEGIDA POR LA LEY)

yoh (1) [name of person authorizing] ah^oo-toh-ree-soh ah (2) [business name] ah dee-bool-gahr lah een-fohr-mah-see^ohn may-dee-kah day
Yo (1) _____ autorizo a (2) _____ a divulgar la información médica de

(3) [name of patient] ah oh-trohs proh-bay-ay-doh-rays day sayr-bee-see^ohs day sah-lood say-goon loh nay-say-sah-ree^oh. tahm-bee^ayn
(3) _____ a otros proveedores de servicios de salud según lo necesario. También,

ah^oo-toh-ree-soh soo dee-bool-gah-see^ohn ah mee kohm-pah-nyee-ah day say-goo-roh may-dee-koh oh kwahl-kee^ayr oh-troh
autorizo su divulgación a mi compañía de seguro médico o cualquier otro

pah-gah-dohr day tayr-say-rohs.
pagador de terceros.

ah-day-mahs kohm-prayn-doh kay tayn-goh ayl day-ray-choh day rray-boh-kahr ay-stah ah^oo-toh-ree-sah-see^ohn ayn kwahl-kee^ayr
Además, comprendo que tengo el derecho de revocar esta autorización en cualquier

moh-mayn-toh. kohm-prayn-doh kay see day-see-doh rray-boh-kahr-lah loh tayn-dray kay ah-sayr pohr ay-skree-toh ee kay kwahl-kee^ayr
momento. Comprendo que si decido revocarla, lo tendré que hacer por escrito y que cualquier

een-fohr-mah-see^ohn dee-bool-gah-dah day ahn-tay-mah-noh noh say bay-rah proh-tay-hee-dah pohr ay-stah rray-boh-kah-see^ohn.
información divulgada de antemano no se verá protegida por esta revocación.

tahm-bee^ayn ayn-tee^ayn-doh kay lah ah^oo-toh-ree-sah-see^ohn day oo-sahr oh dee-bool-gahr lah een-fohr-mah-see^ohn may-dee-kah
También, entiendo que la autorización de usar o divulgar la información médica

ays boh-loon-tah-ree^ah ee noh rray-sool-tah-rah ayn lah day-nay-gah-see^ohn day trah-tah-mee^ayn-toh may-dee-koh.
es voluntaria y no resultará en la denegación de tratamiento médico.

nohm-bray (fah-bohr day ay-skree-beer ayn lay-trahs day mohl-day)
nombre (favor de escribir en letras de molde): _____

feer-mah: *pah-rayn-tay-skoh ahl pah-see^ayn-tay:*
firma: _____ parentesco al paciente: _____

fay-chah:
fecha: _____

Notes

The pronunciation guide need not be learned like the expressions presented in the other chapters. It is only provided to aid the health care provider in assisting iliterate patients or patients who may be visually impaired.

(Spanish version)

CONSENTIMIENTO PARA LA DIVULGACION DE INFORMACION MEDICA
(PROTEGIDA POR LA LEY)

Yo (1) _____ autorizo a (2) _____ a divulgar la información médica

de (3) _____ a otros proveedores de servicios de salud según lo necesario. Tam-

bién, autorizo su divulgación a mi compañía de seguro médico o cualquier otro pagador de ter-

ceros.

Además, comprendo que tengo el derecho de revocar esta autorización en cualquier momento.

Comprendo que si decido revocarla, lo tendré que hacer por escrito y que cualquier información

divulgada de antemano no se verá protegida por esta revocación. También, entiendo que la au-

torización de usar o divulgar la información médica es voluntaria y no resultará en la denegación

de tratamiento médico.

nombre (favor de escribir en letras de molde): _____

firma: _____ parentesco al paciente: _____

fecha: _____

* This page is an example for instructional purposes.

(English version)

MEDICAL INFORMATION RELEASE CONSENT FORM
(PROTECTED BY LAW)

I (1) _____ authorize (2) _____ to release the medical informa-

tion of (3) _____ to other health care providers as deemed necessary. Likewise, I

authorize its release to my insurance company or any other third party payee.

Additionally, I understand that I have the right to revoke this authorization at any time. I under-

stand that should I decide to do so, it must be done in writing and that any information released

prior to this is not protected by this revocation. Also, I understand that the authorization to use

or share medical information is voluntary and will not result in the denial of medical treatment.

name (please print):_____

signature: _____relation to patient: _____

date: _____

* This page is an example for instructional purposes.

Using this form: The (1) requires that the consenting adult write his/her name; (2) requires the name of the medical facility providing treatment; and (3) requires the consenting adult to write the name of the patient whose medical information will be released, which of course, may be the same person.

Practical Activities II

A) Oral Practice

Instructions: With a partner, practice reading the pronunciation guide for the Spanish Medical Information Consent Release Form aloud. Try doing this together first, then take turns reading it aloud to one another seperately. Remember, it does not have to be memorized. Afterwards, prepare the situation given below individually, then present it to one another. Consult past chapters if necessary.

Situation: A patient has returned for a follow-up appointment and the doctor has referred him/her to a specialist. Explain to the patient (s)he has been given a referral and present him/her with the Medical Information Consent Release Form.

Then ask:
- if (s)he can read (response is *no*).
- if you can read the form to him/her (response is *sí*).

(read the form aloud)

- if (s)he understands that consent is given by signing.
- to sign and date the form.

B) Translation

Instructions: Translate the following dialogue between a patient (P) and health care provider (HP). When you have finished, find a partner and compare your translations.

HP — Tenemos los resultados de su procedimiento. Los resultados salieron positivos. Vamos a referirle a un especialista. _____

_____

P — Muy bien. _____

HP — Necesitará programar una cita de inmediato. _____

P — No hay problema. _____

HP — Este es el formulario de consentimiento para la divulgación de información médica. Favor de leerlo. Entonces, fírmelo y féchelo. Tráigamelo cuando haya terminado. _____

_____

P — De acuerdo. *(Patient leaves and comes back a few minutes later.)* _____

HP — ¿Comprende que al firmar este formulario, nos da permiso para compartir la información médica según los términos indicados? _____

_____

P — Sí, comprendo. _____

HP — Llame a este número para programar su cita. Necesitan hacerle unas pruebas adicionales. _____

_____

P — Bien. Gracias, señora. _____

Chapter 16

General Care for Inpatients

Before You Begin

Since family is so important in the Hispanic culture *(familismo)*, the hospitalization of a sick family member is often met with some resistance. This can also be attributed to many other reasons, such as the impersonal medical environment of the Anglo health care system, an unfamiliarity with the foods served, the high cost of hospitalization not to mention fear of a hospital as the place where someone typically goes to die.

Hospitalization also means a temporary seperation from family and loved ones. Therefore, it would not be unlikely that the hospitalized family member be visited by very large groups of people, which may present a problem for other patients and staff. Make sure that signage for visiting hours and the number of patients permitted is visible and in Spanish.

Phrases

English	Pronunciation & Spanish
1. I'm . . .	*soy . . .* Soy . . .
nurse ___.	*ayl an-fayr-**may**-roh / lah ayn-fayr-**may**-rah ___.* el enfermero / la enfermara ___.
doctor ___.	*ayl dohk-**tohr** / lah dohk-**toh**-rah ___.* el doctor / la doctora ___.
2. I am going to show you to your room.	*lay boy ah yay-**bahr** ah soo **kwahr**-toh.* Le voy a llevar a su cuarto.
3. Someone / A family member	***ahl**-ghee^ayn / oon **mee^aym**-broh fah-mee-**lee^ahr*** Alguien / Un miembro familiar
may come with you.	*lay **pway**-day ah-kohm-pah-**nyahr**.* le puede acompañar.
4. Your immediate family / spouse	*soo fah-**mee**-lee^ah een-may-**dee^ah**-tah / pah-**ray**-hah* Su familia inmediata / pareja
may come with you.	***pway**-day ah-kohm-pah-**nyahr**-lay.* puede acompañarle.
5. I need to explain a few things to you.	*lay nay-say-**see**-toh ayk-splee-**kahr** oo-nahs **kwahn**-tahs **koh**-sahs.* Le necesito explicar unas cuántas cosas.

6. This is your . . .
ays soo . . .
Es su . . .

   bed.
   kah-mah.
   cama.

   closet.
   ahr-mah-ree^oh.
   armario.

   bathroom.
   bah-nyoh.
   baño.

   shelf.
   ay-stahn-tay.
   estante.

   nightstand.
   may-see-tah day noh-chay.
   mesita de noche.

7. This is the call bell/buzzer to call
   ay-stay ays ayl teem-bray pah-rah yah-mahr ah
   Este es el timbre para llamar a

   the nurse.
   lah ayn-fayr-may-rah.
   la enfermera.

8. You press it if you need something.
   loh ah-pree^ay-toh see nay-say-see-tah ahl-goh.
   Lo aprieta si necesita algo.

9. Someone will come as soon as possible.
   ahl-ghee^ayn bayn-drah loh mahs prohn-toh poh-see-blay.
   Alguien vendrá lo más pronto posible.

10. This controls the bed.
    ay-stoh kohn-troh-lah lah kah-mah.
    Esto controla la cama.

11. Press this to raise/lower
    ah-pree^ay-tay ay-stoh pah-rah ahl-sahr / bah-hahr
    Apriete esto para alzar / bajar

    (the head of / the foot of) the bed.
    (lah kah-bay-say-rah day / ayl pee^ay day) lah kah-mah.
    (la cabecera de / el pie de) la cama.

12. Please wear slippers / a gown
    fah-bohr day yay-bahr sah-pah-tee-yahs/oo-nah bah-tah
    Favor de llevar zapatillas / una bata

    at all times (when you are not in bed).
    ayn toh-doh moh-mayn-toh (kwahn-doh noh ay-stay ayn kah-mah).
    en todo momento (cuando no esté en cama).

13. Do not get out of bed without assistance.
    noh sah lay-bahn-tay day lah kah-mah seen ah^ee-yoo-dah.
    No se levante de la cama sin ayuda.

14. Do not shift positions without assistance.
    noh say moo^ay-bah ayn lah kah-mah seen ah^ee-yoo-dah.
    No se mueva en la cama sin ayuda.

15. You may only make local
    soh-loh say pway-day ah-sayr yah-mah-dahs
    Sólo se puede hacer llamadas

    calls from this phone.
    loh-kah-lays day ay-stay tay-lay-foh-noh.
    locales de este teléfono.

16. You may make long distance calls from this phone.

*say **pway**-day ah-**sayr** yah-**mah**-dahs day **lahr**-gah dee-**stahn**-see^ah*
Se puede hacer llamadas de larga distancia

*day **ay**-stay tay-**lay**-foh-noh.*
de este teléfono.

17. There is a charge for local calls / long distance calls from this phone/hospital phones.

*say **koh**-brah pohr lahs yah-**mah**-dahs loh-**kah**-lays /*
Se cobra por las llamadas locales /

*yah-**mah**-dahs day **lahr**-gah dee-**stahn**-see^ah **ay**-chahs day*
llamadas de larga distancia hechas de

*ay-stay tay-**lay**-foh-noh / lohs tay-**lay**-foh-nohs dayl oh-spee-**tahl**.*
este teléfono / los teléfonos del hospital.

18. You may purchase a phone card in the gift shop.

*say **pway**-day kohm-**prahr** oo-nah tahr-**hay**-tah tay-lay-**foh**-nee-kah*
Se puede comprar una tarjeta telefónica

*day lah **tee^ayn**-dah day rray-**gah**-lohs*
de la tienda de regalos.

19. To make a local / long distance call, dial nine then wait for the tone. Then dial the number.

*pah-rah ah-**sayr** oo-nah yah-**mah**-dah loh-**kahl** / day **lahr**-gah*
Para hacer una llamada local / de larga

*dee-**stahn**-see^ah **mahr**-kay ayl **noo^ay**-bay ee ay-**spay**-ray ayl **toh**-noh.*
distancia, marque el nueve y espere el tono.

***loo^ay**-goh **mahr**-kay ayl **noo**-may-roh.*
Luego, marque el número.

20. This controls the television.

***ay**-stoh kohn-**troh**-lah lah tay-lay-bee-**see^ohn**.*
Esto controla la televisión.

21. This controls the heating / air conditioning.

***ay**-stoh kohn-**troh**-lah lah kah-lay-fahk-**see^ohn** /*
Esto controla la calefacción /

*ayl **ah^ee**-ray ah-kohn-dee-see^oh-**nah**-doh.*
el aire acondicionado.

22. Please do not change the thermostat.

*fah-**bohr** day noh ahd-hoo-**stahr** ayl tayr-moh-**stah**-toh.*
Favor de no adjustar el termostato.

23. Smoking is not permitted in the hospital.

*noh say payr-**mee**-tay foo-**mahr** ayn ayl oh-spee-**tahl**.*
No se permite fumar en el hospital.

24. You may smoke only in designated areas.

*say **pway**-day foo-**mahr** soh-loh ayn lahs **ah**-ray-ahs day-seeg-**nah**-dahs.*
Se puede fumar sólo en las áreas designadas.

25. You may smoke outside in designated areas only.

*say **pway**-day foo-**mahr** ah-**fway**-rah ee **soh**-loh ayn*
Se puede fumar afuera y sólo en

*lahs **ah**-ray-ahs day-seeg-**nah**-dahs.*
las áreas designadas.

26. They serve . . .

*say **seer**-bay*
Se sirve . . .[1]

  breakfast . . .

*ayl day-sah^ee-**oo**-noh . . .*
el desayuno .

  lunch . . .

*ayl ahl-**moo^ayr**-soh . . .*
el almuerzo . . .

  dinner . . .

*lah **say**-nah . . .*
la cena . . .

27. Here is your . . .

*ah-**kee** . . .*
Aquí . . .

  food.

*ay-**stah** soo koh-**mee**-dah.*
está su comida.

  medicine.

*ay-**stah** soo may-dee-**see**-nah.*
está su medicina.

  belongings.

*ay-**stahn** soos payr-tay-**nayn**-see^ahs.*
están sus pertenencias.

28. A snack is served at . . .

*say **seer**-bay oo-nah may-**ree^ayn**-dah . . .*
Se sirve una merienda . . .[1]

29. You are on a special diet.

*ay-**stah** day **dee^ay**-tah ay-spay-**see^ahl**.*
Está de dieta especial.

30. Please ask that your family

*fah-**bohr** day pay-**deer**-lay ah soo fah-**mee**-lee^ah*
Favor de pedirle a su familia

  not bring you any food.

*kay noh lay **trah^ee**-gah koh-**mee**-dah.*
que no le traiga comida.

31. I will be back . . .

*rray-gray-sah-**ray***
Regresaré . . .

  in to check on you later.

*pah-rah **bayr**-lay mahs **tahr**-day.*
para verle más tarde.

  as fast as I can.

*ayn say-**ghee**-dah.*
en seguida.

32. Do you need assistance / something?

*nay-say-**see**-tah ah^ee-**yoo**-dah / **ahl**-goh?*
¿Necesita ayuda / algo?

33. Do you need to use the restroom?

*nay-say-**see**-tah oo-**sahr** ayl **bah**-nyoh?*
¿Necesita usar el baño?

34. Are you . . .

*tee^**ay**-nay . . .*
¿Tiene . . .

  in pain?

*doh-**lohr**?*
dolor?

  hungry?

ahm-bray?
hambre?

thirsty?	*sayd?* sed?
hot?	*kah-**lohr**?* calor?
cold?	***free**-oh?* frío?

35. Are you (un)comfortable?	*ay-**stah** (een)-**koh**-moh-doh/dah?* ¿Está (in)cómodo/a?[2]

36. Do you need an interpreter?	*nay-say-**see**-tah ah oon een-**tayr**-pray-tay?* ¿Necesita a un intérprete?

37. You need . . .	*nay-say-**see**-tah . . .* Necesita . . .

to rest.	*day-skahn-**sahr**.* descansar.
to relax.	*rray-lah-**hahr**-say.* relajarse.
to calm down.	*kahl-**mahr**-say.* calmarse.
to lie down.	*ah-koh-**stahr**-say.* acostarse.
to sit down.	*sayn-**tahr**-say.* sentarse.
to sit up.	*lay-bahn-**tahr**-say.* levantarse.
to stand up.	*poh-**nayr**-say day pee^ay.* ponerse de pie.
to lie still.	*kay-**dahr**-say een-**moh**-beel.* quedarse inmóvil.
to roll over.	*bohl-**tay**^ahr-say.* voltearse.
to drink this.	*bay-**bayr ay**-stoh.* beber esto.
to eat this.	*koh-**mayr ay**-stoh.* comer esto.
to take this.	*toh-**mahr ay**-stoh.* tomar esto.
to help me (a little).	*ah-yoo-**dahr**-may (oon **poh**-koh).* ayudarme (un poco).

38. Visiting hours are from __ to __.	*lahs oh-rahs day bee-see-tah sohn day __ ah-stah __.* Las horas de visita son de __ hasta __.[1]
39. You may have up to __ visitors at a time.	*pway-day tay-nayr ah-stah __ bee-see-tahn-tays ah lah bays.* Puede tener hasta __ visitantes a la vez.[3]
40. Minors under age __ are not allowed.	*noh say payr-mee-tayn may-noh-rays may-nohs day __ ah-nyohs day ay-dahd.* No se permiten menores menos de __ años de edad.[3]

Notes

[1] Use the information from Chapter 2, #10 to assist you with giving the time at which meals are served. For giving visiting hours follow this model using the information from Chapter 2, #10.

For example: *Las horas de visita son de la una hasta las cuatro de la tarde.*

[2] Use *(in)cómodo* with a male patient and *(in)cómoda* with a female patient.

[3] See **Chapter 18 Numbers**, to complete these phrases as needed.

Practical Activities

A) Oral Practice

Instructions: Prepare the instructions indicated for each situation below. After you have practiced, find a partner and present each set of instructions. As your partner listens, (s)he should make notes that you will use to check his/her comprehension when you have finished your presentations.

Situation 1

Greet a patient, introduce yourself and tell him you will take him to his room. Let him know a family member may come as well. Say you need to explain a few things. Show him his bed, which shelf is his and where the bathroom is located. Show him how to use the buzzer for the nurse as well as the bed control. Also, show him how to adjust the heating and air conditioning. Lastly, tell him what times breakfast, lunch and dinner are served.

Situation 2

A patient has just buzzed you to come to her room. Once you get there, ask her if she needs something. She indicates she is thirsty. After you get her some water, she indicates she would like to make a phone call. You explain she can only make local calls from the phone in her room and that there is charge for them. You tell her she may purchase a phone card in the gift shop. She says thank you. Finally, tell her you will check on her later.

Situation 3

You return to check on a patient and find him agitated. You tell him to calm down and relax. He tries to get out of bed but you tell him not to do so. He begins to calm down a little. You then ask if he is uncomfortable to which he nods yes. He begins to speak rather quickly so you ask if he would like an interpreter. Again, he responds yes. You tell him to lie still and that you will return as fast as you can.

B) Matching

Instructions: Below is a list of words. Write them in the appropriate column in order to create a complete phrase. Check yourself when you are done by looking back in the chapter.

hambre	cama	dolor	la cena	armario
el almuerzo	sed	baño	calor	mesita de noche
estante	el desayuno	frío	una merienda	

Se sirve . . .   ¿Tiene . . .   Es su . . .

Chapter 17

The Body

Parts of the Body

English	Pronunciation & Spanish
the human body	*ayl **kwayr**-poh oo-**mah**-noh* el cuerpo humano
head	*lah kah-**bay**-sah* la cabeza
neck	*ayl **kway**-yoh* el cuello
chest	*ayl **pay**-choh* el pecho
breast	*ayl **say**-noh* el seno
nipple	*ayl pay-**sohn*** el pezón
rib	*lah koh-**stee**-yah* la costilla
stomach	*ayl ay-**stoh**-mah-goh* el estómago
navel	*ayl ohm-**blee**-goh* el ombligo
thigh	*ayl **moo**-sloh* el muslo
knee	*lah rroh-**dee**-yah* la rodilla
calf	*lah pahn-toh-**ree**-yah* la pantorilla
shin	*lah ay-spee-**nee**-yah* la espinilla
ankle	*ayl toh-**bee**-yoh* el tobillo

foot	*ayl pee^ay* **el pie**
toe	*ayl day-doh (dayl pee^ay)* **el dedo (del pie)**
finger	*ayl day-doh* **el dedo**
nail	*lah oo-nyah* **la uña**
chin	*lah bahr-bee-yah* **la barbilla**
hand	*lah mah-noh* **la mano**
wrist	*lah moo-nyay-kah* **la muñeca**
abdomen	*ayl ahb-doh-mayn* **el abdomen**
arm	*ayl brah-soh* **el brazo**
elbow	*ayl koh-doh* **el codo**
face	*lah kah-rah* **la cara**
eye	*ayl oh-hoh* **el ojo**
nose	*lah nah-rees* **la nariz**
mouth	*lah boh-kah* **la boca**
lip	*ayl lah-bee^oh* **el labio**
cheek	*lah may-hee-yah* **la mejilla**
forehead	*lah frayn-tay* **la frente**
eyelid	*ayl pahr-pah-doh* **el párpado**
inner ear	*ayl oh-ee-doh* **el oído**
outer ear	*lah oh-ray-hah* **la oreja**

shoulder	*ayl **ohm**-broh* el hombro
back	*lah ay-**spahl**-dah* la espalda
waist	*lah seen-**too**-rah* la cintura
hip	*lah kah-**day**-rah* la cadera
buttock	*lah **nahl**-gah* la nalga[1]
leg	*lah **pee^ayr**-nah* la pierna
heel	*ayl tah-**lohn*** el talón
coccyx	*ayl **kohk**-seeks* el cóccix[2]
nape	*lah **noo**-kah* la nuca
hamstring	*ayl poh-stay-**ree^ohr** dayl **moo**-sloh* el posterior del muslo
palm	*lah **pahl**-mah* la palma
thorax	*ayl **toh**-rahks* el tórax
groin	*ayl **een**-glay* el ingle
forearm	*ayl ahn-tay-**brah**-soh* el antebrazo
armpit	*lah ahk-**see**-lah* la axila[3]
eyebrow	*lah **say**-hah* la ceja
temple	*ayl see^ayn* el sien

Notes

[1] The plural form of *la nalga*, which is *las nalgas*, may be considered rude by some Hispanics. *Las asentaderas (lahs ah-sayn-tah-**day**-rahs)* is a non-offensive, lower-register term that is used.

[2] Another common term for *cóccix* is *la rabadilla (lah rrah-bah-**dee**-yah)*.

[3] Another common term for *axila* is *el sobaco (ayl soh-**bah**-koh)*.

Internal Organs, Digestive System, and Reproductive Organs

English	Pronunciation & Spanish
internal organs	*lohs **ohr**-gah-nohs een-**tayr**-nohs* los órganos internos
brain	*ayl say-**ray**-broh* el cerebro
spinal cord	*lah **may**-doo-lah ay-spee-**nahl*** la médula espinal
tongue	*lah **layn**-gwah* la lengua
liver	*ayl **ee**-gah-doh* el hígado
esophagus	*ayl ay-**soh**-fah-goh* el esófago
pancreas	*ayl **pahn**-kray-ahs* el páncreas
diaphragm	*ayl dee^ah-**frahg**-mah* el diafragma
spleen	*ayl **bah**-soh* el bazo
lungs	*lohs pool-**moh**-nays* los pulmones
heart	*ayl koh-rah-**sohn*** el corazón
stomach	*ayl ay-**stoh**-mah-goh* el estómago
gallbladder	*lah bay-**see**-koo-lah bee-**lee^ahr*** la vesícula biliar
kidneys	*lohs ree-**nyoh**-nays* los riñones
digestive system	*ayl see-**stay**-mah dee-hay-**stee**-boh* el sistema digestivo
small intestine	*ayl een-tay-**stee**-noh dayl-**gah**-doh* el intestino delgado
large intestine	*ayl een-tay-**stee**-noh **groo^ay**-soh* el intestino grueso

rectum	*ayl **rrayk**-toh* el recto
appendix	*ayl ah-**payn**-dee-say* el apéndice
anus	*ayl **ah**-noh* el ano
reproductive organs	*lohs **ohr**-gah-nohs rray-proh-dook-**tee**-bohs* los óganos reproductivos
fallopian tubes	*lahs **trohm**-pahs* las trompas
ovaries	*lohs oh-**bah**-ree^ohs* los ovarios
uterus	*ayl **oo**-tay-roh* el útero[1]
cervix	*ayl **kway**-yoh dayl **oo**-tay-roh* el cuello del útero
vagina	*lah bah-**hee**-nah* la vagina
seminal vesicle	*ayl bay-**see**-koo-loh say-mee-**nahl*** el vesículo seminal
prostate gland	*lah **proh**-stah-tah* la próstata
urethra	*lah oo-**ray**-trah* la uretra
testicles	*lohs tay-**stee**-koo-lohs* los testículos
scrotum	*ayl ay-**skroh**-toh* el escroto
penis	*ayl **pay**-nay* el pene
prepuce, foreskin	*ayl pray-**poo**-see^oh* el prepucio
vas deferens	*lohs kohn-**dook**-tohs day-fay-**rayn**-tays* los conductos deferentes
bladder	*lah bay-**hee**-gah* la vejiga

Notes

[1]Another term for *el útero* is *la matriz (lah mah-**trees**).*

Chapter 18

The Basics

The Spanish Alphabet[1]

Letter	Pronunciation	Letter	Pronunciation
A	*ah*	O	*oh*
B	*bay*	P	*pay*
C	*say*	Q	*koo*
D	*day*	R	*ay-ray*
E	*ay*	RR	*ay-rray* OR *doh-blay ay-ray*
F	*ay-fay*	S	*ay-say*
G	*hay*	T	*tay*
H	*ah-chay*	U	*oo*
I	*ee*	V	*bay* OR *oo-bay*
J	*hoh-tah*	W	*doh-blay bay* OR *doh-blay oo-bay*
K	*kah*	X	*ay-kees*
L	*ay-lay*	Y	*ee gree^ay-gah*
M	*ay-may*	Z	*say-tah*
N	*ay-nay*	CH[2]	*chay*
Ñ	*ay-nyay*	LL[2]	*ay-yay*

Notes

[1] After practicing the alphabet, have students return to both sections of Chapter 17 and practice spelling the words aloud. Learning to spell in Spanish can be very useful, especially when helping a Spanish-speaker with names, addresses, etc. in English.

[2] These two sounds, once considered letters, no longer form part of the Spanish Alphabet. They have been included since they are commonly used in spelling.

Numbers[1]

Number	Pronunciation	Number	Pronunciation
1	**oo**-noh	40	kwah-**rayn**-tah
2	dohs	50	seen-**kwayn**-tah
3	trays	60	say-**sayn**-tah
4	**kwah**-troh	70	say-**tayn**-tah
5	**seen**-koh	80	oh-**chayn**-tah
6	say^ees	90	noh-**bayn**-tah
7	**see^ay**-tay	100	see^ayn
8	**oh**-choh	101	**see^ayn**-toh **oo**-noh
9	**noo^ay**-bay	150	**see^ayn**-toh seen-**kwayn**-tah
10	dee^ays	200	doh-**see^ayn**-tohs
11	**ohn**-say	300	tray-**see^ayn**-tohs
12	**doh**-say	400	kwah-troh-**see^ayn**-tohs
13	**tray**-say	500	kee-**nee^ayn**-tohs
14	kah-**tohr**-say	600	say-**see^ayn**-tohs
15	**keen**-say	700	say-tay-**see^ayn**-tohs
16	dee^ay-see-**say^ees**	800	oh-choh-**see^ayn**-tohs
17	dee^ay-see-**see^ay**-tay	900	noh-bay-**see^ayn**-tohs
18	dee^ay-see-**oh**-choh	1.000[2]	meel
19	dee^ay-see-**noo^ay**-bay	2.000	dohs meel
20	**bayn**-tay	10.000	dee^ays meel
21	bayn-tee-**oo**-noh	100.000	see^ayn meel
22	bayn-tee-**dohs**	200.000	dohs-**see^ayn**-tohs meel
23	bayn-tee-**trays**	1.000.000	oon mee-**yohn**
24	bayn-tee-**kwah**-troh	10.000.000	dee^ays mee-**yoh**-nays
25	bayn-tee-**seen**-koh	20.000.000	**bayn**-tay mee-**yoh**-nays
26	bayn-tee-**say^ees**	100.000.000	see^ayn mee-**yoh**-nays
27	bayn-tee-**see^ay**-tay	200.000.000	dohs-**see^ayn**-tohs mee-**yoh**-nays
28	bayn-tee-**oh**-choh	1.000.000.000	meel mee-**yoh**-nays[3]
29	bayn-tee-**noo^ay**-bay	2.000.000.000	dohs meel mee-**yoh**-nays[3]
30	**trayn**-tah	0	**say**-roh

Notes

[1] The Spanish spellings have not been included since they are irrelevant for your purposes.

[2] Numbers in Spanish can become quite complicated. Therefore, when working with large sums, it is best to write them out and show the patient. Also, remember, that when writing numbers in Spanish, commas become decimals and decimals become commas; the opposite of the English style of writing numbers.

[3] In American English, *1,000,000,000* would be expressed as *one billion,* which is 10^9. However, in Spanish, this number would be written as *1.000.000.000* and would be expressed as *mil millones,* which literally means *one thousand millions.* The same is true of *2,000,000,000* and so on. The number for *one billion* in Spanish would actually be *1.000.000.000.000* which is 10^{12} and would be expressed as *un billón* which is *one trillion* in American English.

Appendices, Charts, and Images

Making Appointments and Scheduling Follow-up Visits

Instructions: Photocopy this page on cardstock, cut out and laminate. Follow instructions for use as indicated in the NOTES section found in the respective chapter.

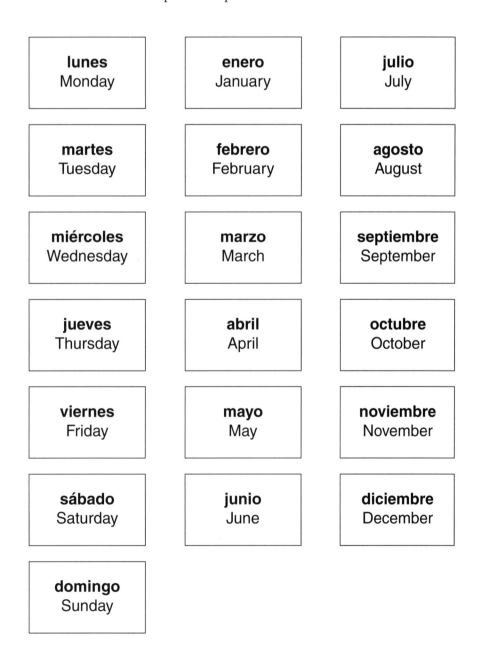

lunes Monday	**enero** January	**julio** July
martes Tuesday	**febrero** February	**agosto** August
miércoles Wednesday	**marzo** March	**septiembre** September
jueves Thursday	**abril** April	**octubre** October
viernes Friday	**mayo** May	**noviembre** November
sábado Saturday	**junio** June	**diciembre** December
domingo Sunday		

Appendix to Chapter 5

Medical History

Personal Medical History

English	Pronunciation & Spanish
chicken pox	*vah-ree-**say**-lah* varicela
diphtheria	*deef-**tay**-ree^ah* difteria
German measles / Rubella	*sah-rahm-**pee^ohn** ah-lay-**mahn** / rroo-**bay**-oh-lah* sarampión alemán / rubéola
measles	*sah-rahm-**pee^ohn*** sarampión
mumps	*pah-**pay**-rahs* paperas
Roseola infantum	*roh-**say**-oh-lah een-fahn-**teel*** roséola infantil
scarlet fever	*ays-kahr-lah-**tee**-nah* escarlatina
viral colds	*kah-**tah**-rohs bee-**rah**-lays* catarros virales
high blood pressure	*pray-**see^ohn** ahl-tah* presión alta (alternate expression)
low blood pressure	*pray-**see^ohn** **bah**-hah* presión baja (alternate expression)

Immunizations and Wellness Testing for School Age Children—Taking Vitals/General Diagnostic Questions

¿Cómo te sientes hoy?

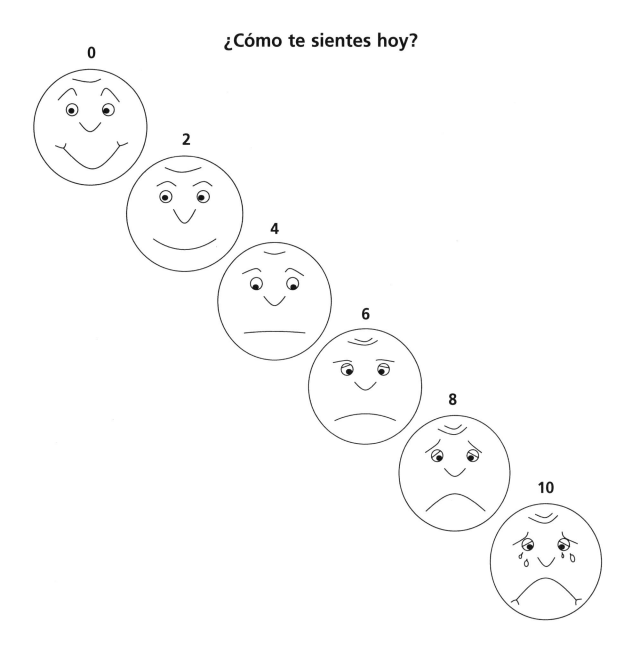

Assessing the Patient's Problem

Preliminary Questions/Pain Assessment

PAIN SCALE / ESCALA DE DOLOR

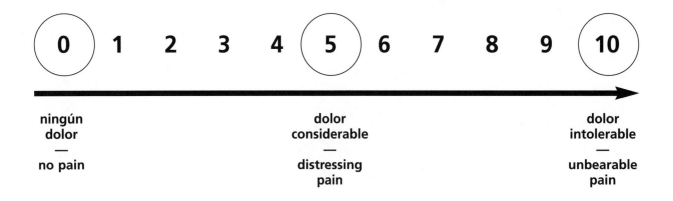

| ningún
dolor
—
no pain | dolor
considerable
—
distressing
pain | dolor
intolerable
—
unbearable
pain |

Assessing the Patient's Problem

The Human Body - Front View / El cuerpo humano - vista anterior

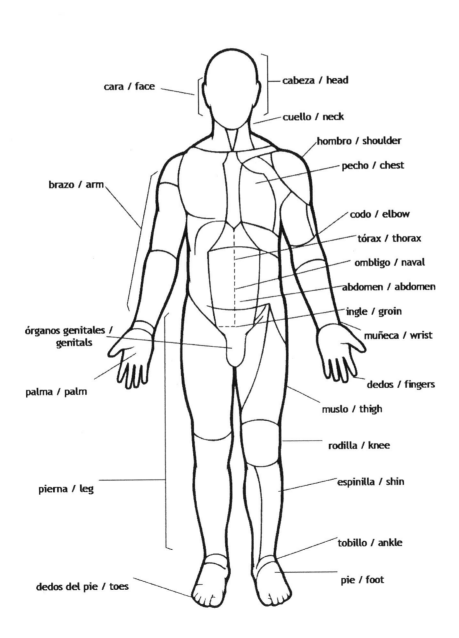

cara / face

cabeza / head

cuello / neck

hombro / shoulder

pecho / chest

brazo / arm

codo / elbow

tórax / thorax

ombligo / naval

abdomen / abdomen

ingle / groin

órganos genitales / genitals

muñeca / wrist

palma / palm

dedos / fingers

muslo / thigh

rodilla / knee

espinilla / shin

pierna / leg

tobillo / ankle

dedos del pie / toes

pie / foot

The Human Body - Rear View / El cuerpo humano - vista posterior

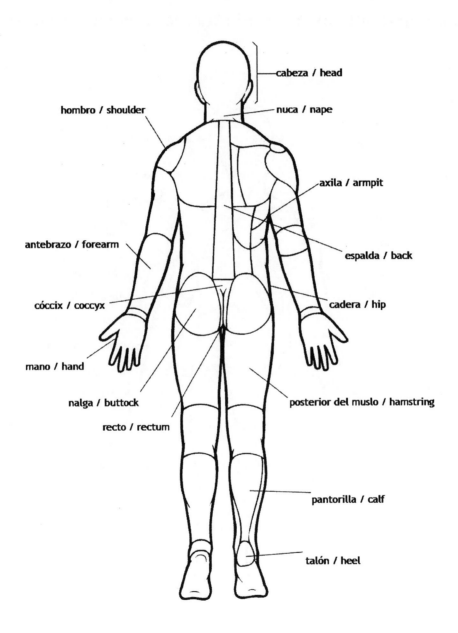

cabeza / head

nuca / nape

hombro / shoulder

axila / armpit

antebrazo / forearm

espalda / back

cóccix / coccyx

cadera / hip

mano / hand

nalga / buttock

recto / rectum

posterior del muslo / hamstring

pantorilla / calf

talón / heel

Assessing the Patient's Problem

Preliminary Questions/Pain Assessment
Common Folk Remedies

English Name	Spanish Name / Pronunciation	Uses
aloe vera	*sah-**bee**-lah* zabila	*burns, cuts and immune system stimulant*
arnica flower tea	*tay day ahr-**nee**-kah* té de arnica	*to treat internal blows, bronchitis, pneumonia, muscle aches*
chamomile	*mahn-sah-**nee**-yah* manzanilla	*diarrhea, menstruation, nausea, colic, anxiety and used as eyewash*
cinnamon tea	*tay day kah-**nay**-lah* té de canela	*digestive aid, coughs, anemia*
corn tassel tea	*tay day **bahr**-bah day* té de barba de *ay-**loh**-tay / mah-**ees*** elote / maíz	*gout, swollen legs, gallstones and kidney problems*
eucalyptus	*ay^oo-kah-**leep**-toh* eucalipto	*asthma, tuberculosis, bronchitis*
fennel tea	*tay day ee-**noh**-hoh* té de hinojo	*vomiting, colic in babies*
garlic	***ah**-hoh* ajo	*high blood pressure, cough syrup, used an an antibiotic*
herb rose tea	*tay day **rroh**-sah day cah-**stee**-yah* té de rosa de castilla	*used as an eyewash for conjunctivitis*
lavender tea	*tay day flohr day sah^oos ee* té de flor de sauz y ***oh**-hahs day ahl-oo-**say**-mah* hojas de alhucema	*fever, measles*

lead/mercury oxides	*ah-sahr-**kohn** / **gray**-tah* azarcón / greta	*teething*
orange blossom tea	*tay day ah-sah-**ahr*** té de azahar	*nerve and heart conditions*
oregano	*oh-**ray**-gah-noh* orégano	*worms, menstrual problems*
parsley tea	*tay day ohs-ah* té de osha	*kidney infections*
rosemary tea	*tay day rroh-**may**-roh* té de romero	*stimulates digestion and regulates menstruation*
sage	*sah-**lee**-bah* saliva	*diabetes, hair loss*
sarsaparilla tea	*tay day koh-kohl-**may**-kah* té de cocolmeca	*gout, syphilis, psoriasis, kidney problems, rheumatism*
trumpet flowers	*troh-nah-**doh**-rah* tronadora	*adult onset diabetes, chickenpox*
wild marjoram tea	*tay day oh-**ray**-gah-noh* té de orégano	*intestinal infections, regulates menstruation*

Assessing the Patient's Problem

Diagnostic Questions - Cardiopulmonary System
FREQUENCY CHART / GRAFICO DE FRECUENCIA

WHEN? *¿Cuándo?*	HOW OFTEN? *¿Cuántas veces?*	HOW MANY DAYS? *¿Por cuántos días?*
siempre / always	1	1
—	—	—
al día / a day	2	2
—	—	—
cada dos días / every two days	3	3
—	—	—
a la semana / a week	4	4
—	—	—
cada dos semanas / every two weeks	5	5
—	—	—
al mes / a month	6	6
—	—	—
cada dos o tres meses / every two or three months	7	7
—	—	—
cada seis o siete meses / every six or seven months	8	8
—	—	—
al año / a year	9	9
	—	—
	10	10
	—	—
	más de 10 / more than 10	*más de 10 /* more than 10

Bibliography

"A Systematic Approach to Health Improvement." *Healthy People 2010*. 7 Sept. 2006
     <http://www.healthypeople.gov/document/html/uih/uih_2.htm>.
About: Spanish Language. Ed. Gerald Erichsen. 2006. 31 July 2006
     <http://spanish.about.com/>
"About Minority Health." *Office of Minority Health*. Centers for Disease Control and Prevention. 3 Sept. 2006
     <http://www.cdc.gov/omh/AMH/AMH.htm>.
Buckel, Mike. Group interview. 9 Aug. 2006.
Childhood Immunization. Medline Plus. U.S. National Library of Medicine and the National Institutes of
     Health. 15 Sept. 2006
     <http://www.nlm.nih.gov/medlineplus/immunization.html>.
Clínica de Ojos Dr. Nano. 15 Sept. 2006
     <http://www.clinano.com.ar/folletos/lae.htm>
Clutter, Ann W. and Ruben D. Nieto. "Understanding the Hispanic Culture." The Ohio State University Fact
     Sheet. Ohio State University Extension. 25 Aug. 2006
     <http://ohioline.osu.edu/hyg-fact/5000/5237.html>.
"Consejos para padres con hijos adolescentes". 2001-2004. GuíasJuvenil.com. 15 Sept. 2006
     <http://www.guiajuvenil.com/index.htm>.
Cuadros, Paul. "Hispanic Workers Health Needs are Overwhelming Southern Poultry Towns." *The APF Re-
     porter* 19.4 (2001). 16 Sept. 2006
     <http://www.aliciapatterson.org/APF1904/Cuadros/Cuadros.html>.
Freeman, Kris S. "Latino Culture and Health Communication." 9 Sept. 2006
     <staff.washington.edu/kfreeman/Freeman-STC2002-Latinohealthcom.PDF>.
Generic Name List. NeedyMeds.com. 20 Sept. 2006
     <http://www.needymeds.com/generic_list.taf>
"Health care & Hispanics: Understanding Cultural Differences is the Key." *Hispanic Tips*. 2005. Niche New
     Media. 14 June 2006
     <http://hispanictips.com/2005/10/27/health care-us-Hispanics-understanding-cultural-differences-is-the-
     key/>
Healthwise Handbook. Kaiser Permanente. 10 Sept. 2006
     <http://www.permanente.net/homepage/handbook/healthwisehandbook/chapter_index/ch_index_
     spanish.htm>.
"Immunization." *Medline Plus*. U.S. National Library of Medicine and the National Institutes of Health. 15
     Sept. 2006
     <http://www.nlm.nih.gov/medlineplus/immunization.html>.
"Información en español". *AHRQ: Agency for Health care Research and Quality*. United States Department of
     Health and Human Services. 15 Aug. 2006
     <http://www.ahrq.gov/consumer/espanoix.htm>.
Kelz, Rochelle K. *Conversational Spanish for Health Professionals*. 3rd ed. Canada: Delmar Publishers, 1999.
Lebrado, Jarvis. *Spanish for Medical Personnel*. 5th ed. Lexington, D. C. Heath and Company, 1996.

Leigh-Martinez, Daniel. "Traditional Latino Medicines: The Newly Discovered Alternative Medicine." 29 Aug. 2006
    <http://www.public.asu.edu/~squiroga/leigh.HTM>.

Lusk, Sally. Group interview. 9 Aug. 2006.

McElroy, Onyria H. and Lola L. Grabb. *Spanish-English English-Spanish Medical Dictionary*. 2nd ed. United States of America: Little, Brown and Company, 1996.

Mikkelson, Holly. "The Art of Working with Interpreters: A Manual for Health Care Professionals." Acebo. 15 Aug. 2006
    <http://www.acebo.com/papers/artintrp.htm>

Nack, Pamela. Group interview. 9 Aug. 2006.

"Pain Level Chart." *Home and Care Hospice Services*. Holy Redeemer Health System. 1999-2005. 15 Sept. 2006
    <http://www.holyredeemer.com/page.php?id=389>.

"Remedios Caseros". *Tu Abuela*. 3 Sept. 2006 <http://www.tuabuela.com/modificaciones/indexremedios.htm>.

"Statistics." *HIV Among Hispanics*. 2006. Centers for Disease Control and Prevention. 10 Oct. 2006
    <http://www.cdc.gov/hiv/resources/factsheets/hispanic.htm>.

Tu Pediatra.com. Ed. Dr. Meyer Magarici. 20 Sept. 2006 <http://www.tupediatra.com/>.

Twenty of the Most Frequently Asked Questions about the Hispanic Community. 12 Aug. 2006
    <http://lacc.fiu.edu/events_outreach/teacher_training/faq.pdf>.

CD-ROM Contents

The audio files on the enclosed CD-ROM are in the MP-3 format, and can be played on MP-3 players, most computers, and many CD players.